# Headache

## Egilius L.H. Spierings, M.D., Ph.D.

*Consultant in Neurology, Brigham and Women's*
*Hospital; Lecturer in Neurology, Harvard*
*Medical School, Boston*

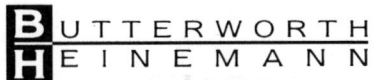

Boston  Oxford  Johannesburg  Melbourne  New Delhi  Singapore

**Library of Congress Cataloging-in-Publication Data**
Spierings, Egiluis L. H., 1953-
    Headache / Egilius L.H. Spierings.
        p.    cm. -- (The most common complaints)
    Includes bibliographical references and index.
    ISBN 0-7506-7128-9 (alk. paper)
    1. Headache.  I. Title.  II. Series.
    [DNLM: 1. Headache. WL 342 S755h 1998]
RB 128.S65 1998
616.8'491--dc21
DNLM/DLC
for Library of Congress                                98-3398
                                                        CIP

**British Library Cataloguing-in-Publication Data**
A catalogue record for this book is available from the British Library.

The publisher offers special discounts on bulk orders of this book.
For information, please contact:
Manager of Special Sales                For information on all
Butterworth–Heinemann                    Butterworth–Heinemann
225 Wildwood Avenue                      publications available,
Woburn, MA  01801-2041                   contact our World Wide Web
Tel: 781-904-2500                        home page at:
Fax: 781-904-2620                        http://www.bh.com

10 9 8 7 6 5 4 3 2 1

Printed in the United States of America

*For Malina, in gratitude for two decades
of love and support*

# Contents

## PART THREE: CHRONIC HEADACHE

# Tables

# Preface

Headache is a common complaint in medical practice. It is a complaint often dreaded because of the great number and variety of etiologies headache covers. Headache can be caused by a condition as benign as an upper respiratory infection or as deadly as a subarachnoid hemorrhage. Headache can also be deceptive in its presentation, especially in the elderly, in whom it can lead to blindness (temporal arteritis) or death (subdural hematoma) before the nature of the problem is determined. In chronic headache, whether present intermittently (migraine or cluster headache) or continuously (chronic daily headache), treatment is often a challenge. Hence, headache can be a source of tremendous frustration for the physician *and* patient alike.

This book assists the medical practitioner with an overview of headache that is both comprehensive and concise. The book is structured around case studies to facilitate recognition of the headache conditions discussed. The approach is practical and draws heavily on my experience in diagnosing and treating headache patients. I also draw on the knowledge imparted to me through extensive training with John R. Graham (1909–1990). Dr. Graham was a physician and educator who has been referred to as the "father of headache management." With regard to headache mechanisms, I am, through Dr. Graham, greatly influenced by Harold G. Wolff (1898–1962). Dr. Wolff was responsible for the most comprehensive research in headache, and therefore can be rightly called the "father of headache research." For my understanding of the neurologic and neurosurgical aspects of headache, I am indebted to my teachers in these respective areas: Arthur Staal, M.D., and Reinder Braakman, M.D.

I also acknowledge with pleasure the help of my friends and colleagues, Laurens Mulder, M.D., and David Coddon, M.D., who kindly reviewed the manuscript. The manuscript was converted into this handsome book by the skillful hands at Butterworth–Heinemann and Silverchair Science + Communications. Last, but certainly not least, I thank my wife, Malina, and my children, Sven and Natalia, for tolerating my preoccupation with medicine in general and with headache in particular.

E.L.H.S.

# Introduction

In the absence of injury, the head hurts more often than any other part of the body. Seventy to 80% of the population, men and women alike, experience headache. Fifty percent of the population experience headache at least once per month, 15% at least once per week, and 5% daily.

As a result of its high prevalence, headache is a common complaint in medical practice. It is the second most common complaint in primary care practice, reported by 28% of patients.[1] It follows fatigue, which is reported by 29% of patients.

Headache is generally divided into three categories on the basis of intensity: mild, moderate, and severe. The rating of the intensity level depends on the extent to which the headache interferes with the ability to function. Mild headaches do not interfere with the ability to function, moderate headaches interfere with the ability to function but do not require bed rest, and severe headaches are incapacitating and require bed rest.

Moderate and severe headaches are twice as common in women as in men. The reason for this is largely that women have an estrogen cycle related to menses. The menstrual cycle is a common precipitant of moderate and severe headaches in women. Moderate headaches occur in 13% of men and 23% of women; severe headaches occur in 6% and 12%, respectively.[2]

Headaches are not only gender-dependent but also age-dependent. The prevalence of headache sharply increases during the second decade of life, in men and women alike. It then levels off until the age of 40–50 years, after which it gradually decreases.

Headaches, independent of their frequency of occurrence, are familial. The strongest positive family history is found for patients' parents, of whom one or both are affected in 60% of cases.[3] The mother is affected almost twice as frequently as the father (46% versus 26%). The positive family history is the same for migraine as it is for headaches in general. This suggests that familial occurrence of headache is also independent of headache intensity.

In medical practice, headache presents itself as an *acute, subacute,* or *chronic* condition. Acute headache is generally severe in intensity and usually presents in the emergency room. Subacute and chronic headaches, on the other hand, present in the office. Diagnostic considerations depend largely on the presentation of the headache. Therefore, the differential diagnosis of headache is discussed in this book in three sections based on the three presentations. It is important to remember, however, that whatever the presentation, headache is *always* a valid complaint. It should *always* be investigated seriously and *never* considered merely a product of the imagination.

## REFERENCES

1. Nederlands Instituut voor Onderzoek van de Eerstelijnsgezonheidszorg (NIVEL). Nationale Studie naar Ziekten en Verrichtingen in de Huisartsenpraktijk, een Caleidoscoop. Utrecht, The Netherlands: NIVEL, 1997.
2. Goldstein M, Chen TC. The epidemiology of disabling headache. Adv Neurol 1982;33:377–390.
3. Messinger HB, Spierings ELH, Vincent AJP, Lebbink J. Headache and family history. Cephalalgia 1991;11:13–18.

# Overview of Headache

In medical practice, headache can be acute, sub-acute, or chronic, depending on the length of time it has been present, either intermittently or continuously: The acute headache has been present for hours or days, the subacute headache for days or weeks, and the chronic headache for months or years. In the context of headache, the term *chronic* is also used to refer to the daily or almost daily occurrence of headaches, as in chronic daily headache. To make matters even more confusing, it is also used to refer to the occurrence of headaches without remission, as opposed to episodic (with remission). The latter use of *chronic* is found in chronic (as opposed to episodic) cluster headache.

---

## ETIOLOGY

---

The length of time that headaches have been present can give direction about which etiologies to consider. With acute headache, an important question to address is whether similar headaches have occurred before.

### Headache Pattern

Certain chronic headache conditions are characterized by the recurrence of headache with relatively long headache-free intervals (e.g., migraine or cluster headache). Sometimes, a headache is preceded by similar headaches of lesser intensity, such as the so-called *sentinel headaches* in subarachnoid hemorrhage. When an acute headache is preceded by similar headaches, it is important to ascertain that the current headache is indeed similar to the preceding ones. A headache that is significantly different from prior headaches can have a different etiology. For example, a patient with migraine can have a different headache from the normal migraine, one that may signify structural neurologic illness. The following case study illustrates this pattern.

---

A 47-year-old woman presented with headache and difficulty speaking. The symptoms started 2 weeks before consultation, with the onset of menstruation. She had a history of headaches going back to her teenage years. The headaches always occurred with menstruation and lasted 1–2 days. They were severe in intensity and were associated with nausea, vomiting, photophobia, and phonophobia. The headaches were usually located in the right temple and forehead. The present headache started, as usual, with menstruation, but it was generalized in location and, although as intense, it was not associated with nausea or vomiting. Also, the headache had continued long beyond its usual duration. On examination, she was somewhat slow mentally, and there was a slight hesitation in her speech. Her fundi revealed edema of the optic disks (papilledema). The reflexes were brisker on the left than on the right, and the plantar reflex was pathologic on the left. Computed tomography showed marked displacement of the midline structures to the right (Fig. 1-1). Angiography revealed this to be due to a large subdural hematoma on the left (Fig. 1-2). After evacuation of the hematoma, the headache and speech disturbance subsided. The patient then remembered that 2 weeks before the onset of the headache, she was hit in the head by the boom of her sailboat.

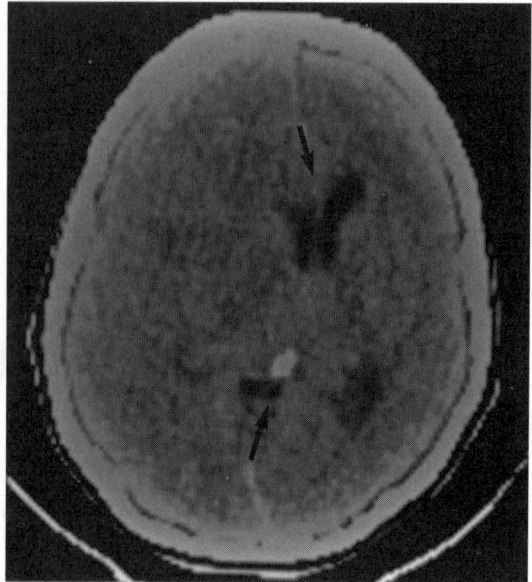

**Figure 1-1.** Computed tomogram with contrast shows an isodense subdural hematoma on the left, with midline structures shifted to the right (arrows).

## Acute Headache

When an acute, severe headache is preceded by similar headaches, it is reasonable to consider migraine as a diagnosis. Without such a prior history, how-

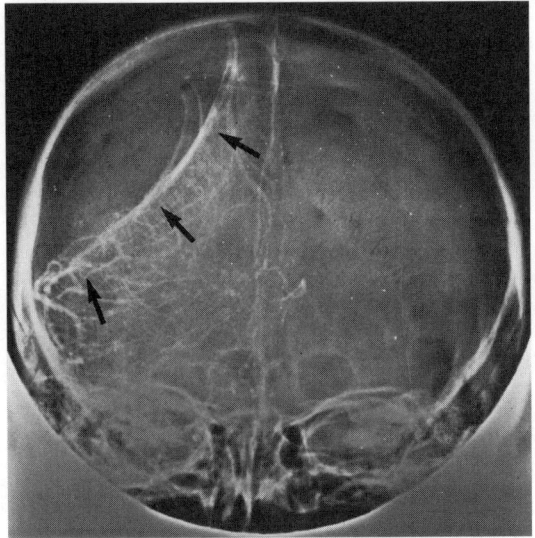

**Figure 1-2.** Cerebral angiogram shows (left) a displacement of blood vessels away from the skull (arrows), consistent with a large subdural hematoma (same patient as in Fig. 1-1).

ever, one must be very careful. I once made this mistake when I saw a middle-aged man with headache in the emergency room. He had had a severe generalized headache for several days, associated with nausea and vomiting. A language barrier prevented me from obtaining accurate information on the mode of onset of the headache.

In evaluating acute headache, it is very important to know how long it took for the headache to develop. Usually, I ask the patient how long it took for the headache to build to its maximum intensity. I try to obtain as precise an answer as possible—that is, in seconds, such as with a blow to the head, or in minutes or hours. A headache that starts in a matter of seconds should raise suspicion of an intracranial hemorrhage. A buildup to maximum intensity in minutes is typical of cluster headache, whereas a migraine headache generally takes hours to develop.

In the case of the man in the emergency room, I was not able to obtain this crucial information. I proceeded with the neurologic examination, which was entirely normal, including the fundi. I subsequently concluded that it was a migraine headache. The next day, the patient came back with the same headache. Computed tomography was performed, revealing a hematoma in a pituitary adenoma.

Apart from intracranial hemorrhage, it is also always important to consider meningitis in the evaluation of acute, severe headache. Fever is usually present in these cases, but the temperature may have to be measured to determine the presence of fever. Hypertensive encephalopathy can also present as acute, severe headache, and diagnosis requires measuring the blood pressure. The neurologic examination may reveal papilledema in either case but may otherwise be normal.

## Subacute Headache

The conditions to consider in subacute headache, in which the headache has been present for days or weeks are, to a great extent, dependent on the age of the patient. Subdural hematoma, temporal arteritis, and ophthalmic zoster are mostly conditions of the elderly. In the younger population, cerebral tumor is important to consider, but, except in children, it is usually associated with neurologic symptoms or signs. Pseudotumor cerebri, also referred to as *benign* or *idiopathic intracranial hypertension*, may manifest as a cerebral tumor—that is, with headache and papilledema but without localizing symptoms or signs.

## Chronic Headache

In the adult population younger than age 50–60 years, chronic headache conditions are the most common. The headaches have been present for months or years and sometimes even decades. They are often intermittent but can be continuous. The latter pattern characterizes a significant number of people (5% of the population experience daily head-aches). Many intermittent headaches are mild in intensity and respond to nonprescription analgesics. Patients often refer to them as *regular headaches*; the International Headache Society classifies them as *episodic tension-type headaches*. They used to be called *muscle-contraction* or *tension headaches*. The following is a typical case of episodic tension-type or muscle-contraction headache.

---

A 61-year-old woman has had headaches for as long as she can remember. The headaches occur twice per week on average. They start during the day and are brought on by rushing around, among other factors. The headaches are mild in intensity and last for 1–3 hours. They are located across the forehead and are sometimes associated with mild tightness of the neck and shoulder muscles.

---

## Eyestrain Headache

Although it is disputed by many ophthalmologists, regular headaches can also be caused by eyestrain. The problem in such cases is relative weakness of the muscles of accommodation. It manifests in headache rather than in blurring of near vision, which is usually the case when the weakness develops later in life. On further questioning, however, these generally young patients may indicate blurring of vision with prolonged reading, working at a computer terminal, or watching television (latent hyperopia). They may also experience momentary blurring of distant vision after prolonged near-vision activity, which is referred to as pseudomyopia. Another feature that often characterizes these patients is excellent distant vision—they tend to be the first in the car to read a road sign—and extreme sensitivity to light, requiring them to wear sunglasses wherever they go. The following case study illustrates regular or tension-type headaches caused by eyestrain, or asthenopia.

---

A 27-year-old woman has had headaches since she went back to school 2 years ago. The headaches occur twice per week on average and last for 15–20 minutes. The headaches are mild in intensity and feel like a tightness across the forehead. They are brought on by prolonged reading or working at a computer terminal. Under these circumstances, she may also experience blurring of vision. Sometimes her vision is blurred when she looks into the distance after prolonged near vision. Focusing her eyes on a distant object may help to relieve the headaches. The headaches tend to dissipate quickly anyway with cessation of near-vision activity. She is always sensitive to light and has to wear sunglasses whenever she goes outside. The headaches improved with the use of low-strength magnifiers for near vision.

## Sinus Headache

Some patients refer to their regular headaches as *sinus headaches* because of the location of pain over the sinuses—that is, across the forehead. These patients take nonprescription sinus medications for the headaches with relief. Sinus headaches are probably so-called *sinus-vacuum headaches*, caused by obstruction of the ostia to the sinuses. The condition is also referred to as *barosinusitis* and results from swelling of the nasal mucosa that is triggered by allergies, exposure to smells or odors, damp weather, and so on. The pain is typically located in the cheeks or in the center of the forehead and bridge of the nose. The following is a typical case of sinus headache or barosinusitis.

A 44-year-old woman has had headaches for 5 years. The headaches occur in the fall and sometimes also in the spring. They are usually present on awakening in the morning, last 1–2 hours, and are relieved by the use of a corticosteroid nasal spray. They are located in the cheeks and in the bridge of the nose. The headaches feel like a pressure and are associated with nasal congestion. They can also be brought on by exposure to a strong chemical odor or strong perfume.

## MEDICAL CONSULTATION

Patients with episodic tension-type or sinus-vacuum headaches generally do not seek medical advice because of the relief they receive from nonprescription medications. When the headaches become more frequent and merge into what has been referred to as *chronic daily headache*, however, the patient may knock on your door. In a study of patients with at least 10 days of tension headache per month, almost two-thirds experienced daily headaches.[1] This suggests that when headaches increase to a frequency of two or three times per week, they tend to progress rapidly to daily or almost daily occurrence.

Another reason that patients with chronic headache conditions seek medical advice is a lack of response to nonprescription medications. This generally occurs when the headaches become more intense, and their intensity affects the functioning of the stomach. The stomach dysfunction impairs the absorption of medications taken by mouth, which is invariably the route of administration of nonprescription medications. Migraine is a typical example of a chronic headache condition in which this occurs (see Chapter 19).

## SEVERE HEADACHE

Apart from migraine, severe headaches are also seen in cluster headache. In this chronic condition, the headaches evade effective treatment with nonprescription medications, not only because of their intensity but also because of their rapid onset and relatively short duration. Severe headaches are also encountered in chronic daily headache, in which they occur as a result of further progression of the headaches after they have become daily and continuous and take up all available time. Severe headaches also occur in chronic daily headache when the condition develops out of migraine as a result of a gradual increase in frequency of the migraine headaches and a progressive interposition of migraine headaches with tension-type headaches (see Chapter 14).

### Chronic Daily Headache

Patients with chronic daily headache have daily or almost daily headaches. The headaches may have been daily from the onset or may have become daily after initially intermittent tension-type or migraine headaches (see Chapter 21). Patients often do not mention the daily or almost daily occurrence of their headaches, and this is something that must be specifically asked about. It is especially important to ask this question of patients with frequent migraine headaches. It is virtually impossible to have migraine headaches on a weekly basis without having daily or almost daily headaches.

## Intermittent Headache

As stated in Medical Consultation, when intermittent headaches are mild, they are generally relieved by nonprescription medications. Patients tend not to seek medical advice for these headaches unless they occur frequently (i.e., daily or almost daily). When the headaches are more intense and do not respond to nonprescription medications, patients seek medical advice regardless of their frequency. The diagnostic considerations are then largely determined by the temporal pattern of the headaches—that is, their frequency and duration. In migraine, the headaches last hours to days and often occur on a monthly basis, typically once or twice per month. In cluster headache, they last 1–2 hours and occur daily for weeks or months when episodic, and for longer than a year when chronic.

## **REFERENCE**

1. Langemark M, Olesen J, Poulsen DL, Bech P. Clinical characterization of patients with chronic tension headache. Headache 1988;28:590–596.

# PART ONE

# Acute Headache

C H A P T E R   T W O

# Clinical Approach to Acute Headache

Headache not caused by trauma is responsible for 1–2% of visits to the emergency room.[1] Men and women are equally represented, and 80% of the patients are between 15 and 54 years of age. Muscle-contraction headache is the most common diagnosis (32%), followed by migraine (22%) and upper respiratory infection (12%) (Table 2-1). The following diagnoses each account for 5% or less of nontraumatic headache in the emergency room: sinusitis, hypertension, gastroenteritis, cerebral tumor, and cervical spine degeneration. Apart from cerebral tumor, the neurologic causes of headache (i.e., subarachnoid hemorrhage, meningitis, ophthalmic zoster, temporal arteritis, and subdural hematoma) each account for less than 1%. Headache as it is pre-

**Table 2-1. Diagnosis of nontraumatic headache in the emergency room (n = 485)**

| Diagnosis | Percentage of patients |
|---|---|
| Muscle-contraction headache | 32 |
| Migraine | 22 |
| Upper respiratory infection | 12 |
| Sinusitis | 5 |
| Hypertension | 4 |
| Gastroenteritis | 3 |
| Cerebral tumor | 3 |
| Cervical spine degeneration | 2 |

Source: Adapted from MJ Leicht. Non-traumatic headache in the emergency department. Ann Emerg Med 1980;9:404–409.

sented in the emergency room also may be encountered during house visits.

## EXAMINATION OF THE PATIENT WITH ACUTE HEADACHE

What is the *general impression* of the patient: sick, feverish, drowsy, irritable, confused? Obtain the *temperature*, *blood pressure*, and *pulse rate* first, and then carefully examine the neck for *meningeal irritation*. The neck examination should be done gently, with the back of the patient's head resting in the palms of the examiner's hands. The patient's neck is first rotated to each side, after which it is bent forward so that the chin touches the chest. While the patient's neck is being bent forward, the patient's face is watched for indications of pain and the legs for signs of flexion. Limited forward flexion of the neck is significant only when rotation of the neck is intact. Otherwise, it is merely an indication of tightness of the neck muscles, which many headache patients experience, especially during the presence of headache (see Chapter 13).

## DIAGNOSTIC CONSIDERATIONS

The presence of fever suggests upper respiratory infection, sinusitis, or gastroenteritis as possible causes of the headache (Table 2-2). Each of these conditions comes with specific symptoms, such as sore throat, cough, nasal discharge, postnasal drip, nausea, vomiting, or diarrhea.

The combination of fever with meningeal irritation raises suspicion of meningitis, either viral or bacterial. In this case, lumbar puncture should be performed once cerebral involvement (e.g., encephalitis, cerebral abscess) has been excluded by neurodiagnostic imaging (e.g., computed tomography or magnetic resonance imaging).

Meningeal irritation without fever may indicate subarachnoid hemorrhage, for which neurodiagnos-

**Table 2-2. Differential diagnosis of acute, severe headache**

With fever but without meningeal irritation
    Upper respiratory infection
    Sinusitis
    Gastroenteritis
With fever *and* meningeal irritation
    Viral or bacterial meningitis
With meningeal irritation but without fever
    Subarachnoid hemorrhage

tic imaging (computed tomography without contrast) should be performed. If the results of imaging are negative, it should be followed by lumbar puncture.

Cerebral tumor is a cause of subacute headache, but it may present with acute headache when the tumor is complicated by hemorrhage. This is seen, in particular, with chromophobe adenomas of the pituitary gland and cerebral metastases of malignant melanoma. With hemorrhage into a pituitary adenoma, there may be no other symptoms than severe headache (see Chapter 1). Therefore, it is not possible to make this diagnosis without performing neurodiagnostic imaging. Generally, with cerebral tumors, neurologic symptoms are present or abnormalities can be found on the neurologic examination.

Ophthalmic zoster, temporal arteritis, and subdural hematoma should be considered in patients older than age 60 years with subacute headache. Temporal arteritis is generally associated with a significantly elevated sedimentation rate of 50 mm per hour or higher. Therefore, it is important to perform this simple test in *all* patients age 60 years or older who present with headache. Tension-type headache and migraine are chronic headache conditions. Hence, if they are diagnosed as acute headache, there must be a prior history of similar headaches.

Cerebral tumor, ophthalmic zoster, temporal arteritis, and subdural hematoma as causes of headache are discussed in detail in Part II of this book, together with pseudotumor cerebri. Meningitis, subarachnoid hemorrhage, and hypertensive encephalopathy as causes of acute headache are discussed in the remaining chapters of Part I.

## REFERENCE

1. Leicht MJ. Non-traumatic headache in the emergency department. Ann Emerg Med 1980;9:404–409.

# Meningitis

A 17-year-old man presents with severe headache in the emergency room. The headache started the previous day around noon. It gradually built in intensity but was not severe until it woke him out of sleep at 2 AM. The headache is located across the forehead and is throbbing in nature. It is associated with photophobia, nausea, vomiting, and diarrhea. He also feels off balance and cannot walk straight. The headache is made worse by coughing and bending over, but ice applied to the forehead makes it somewhat better. He does not have a fever but relates that he felt hot and cold the day before. His sister was sick with the flu a week earlier. On examination, he is clearly sick with headache and gastrointestinal upset. His fundi cannot be examined because of

extreme sensitivity to light. It is slightly difficult to
bend his neck forward. A lumbar puncture shows
clear and colorless fluid under a normal pressure.
The spinal fluid contains 380 cells per µl, of which
90% are lymphocytes, indicating viral meningitis.

## INCIDENCE AND ETIOLOGY

The incidence of meningitis in the United States is
estimated at 10–20 cases per 100,000 population per
year. Children younger than age 5 years account for
70% of the cases. About half of the cases are caused
by a bacterial infection, usually involving *Haemophilus
influenzae*, *Neisseria meningitidis* (petechiae should be
looked for), or *Streptococcus pneumoniae*. The infection is generally hematogenic, and the site of entry of
the organisms into the blood is usually the upper respiratory tract. When not caused by a bacterial infection, the meningitis is usually viral. The viruses
involved are usually enteroviruses, followed by the
mumps virus, arboviruses, and herpes simplex virus.

## PRESENTATION AND DIAGNOSIS

Meningitis develops acutely over hours or days.
It may or may not be preceded by a respiratory or

gastrointestinal illness. Severe, bilateral headache associated with photophobia, nausea, and vomiting is its main presentation. When the cause is bacterial, altered sensorium with drowsiness, disorientation, and confusion is common. Fever and signs of meningeal irritation are found in 80% of meningitis cases. The diagnosis is made through lumbar puncture and analysis of spinal fluid, which should be performed in *every* suspected case.

## BACTERIAL VERSUS VIRAL MENINGITIS

Patients with bacterial meningitis are usually much sicker than those with viral meningitis. However, a distinction between the two can only be made by analyzing the spinal fluid (Table 3-1).

In bacterial meningitis, the cell count generally exceeds 1,000 per μl, with 90% polymorphonuclear leukocytes. The protein level is usually significantly elevated and the glucose level decreased. In viral meningitis, the cell count is generally less than 1,000 per μl, with the cells being mostly lymphocytes. Protein and glucose levels are normal. If no distinction can be made and the patient is *not* seriously ill, the spinal fluid should be re-examined

**Table 3-1. Spinal fluid analysis in viral and bacterial meningitis**

| Type | Analysis |
|------|----------|
| Viral | Cell count <1,000/μl |
| | Mostly lymphocytes |
| | Protein and glucose levels normal |
| Bacterial | Cell count >1,000/μl |
| | Mostly polymorphonuclear leukocytes |
| | Protein level significantly elevated |
| | Glucose level decreased |

after 6 hours. Bacterial meningitis is treated with antibiotics; treatment of viral meningitis is symptomatic only.

# Subarachnoid Hemorrhage

A 56-year-old woman is brought to the emergency room by her husband because of severe headache. The headache started the night before during intercourse. She suddenly grabbed her head and was dazed for a short time. After taking some pain medication, she slept all night, but in the morning, her husband had difficulty waking her. The headache was still severe, and she vomited several times. He had to support her down the stairs because she could not see the steps very well. On examination, she looks sick and is somewhat drowsy. She complains of severe headache with extreme pressure on the eyes. Her temperature is normal; the fundi show normal optic disks and no bleeding. Forward flexion

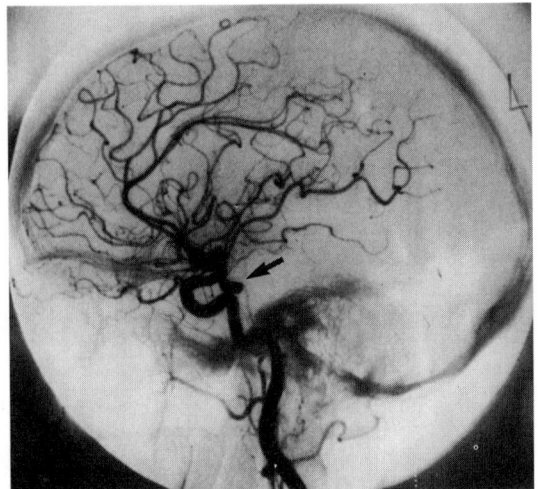

**Figure 4-1.** Cerebral angiogram shows an aneurysm originating from the posterior communicating artery close to its origin from the internal carotid artery (arrow).

of the neck is severely limited, but rotation is intact. Computed tomography is negative. A lumbar puncture reveals hemorrhagic fluid, which is yellow after centrifugation. Angiography shows the source of the bleeding to be an aneurysm of the left posterior communicating artery (Fig. 4-1).

## INCIDENCE AND ETIOLOGY

The annual incidence of subarachnoid hemorrhage in the United States is estimated at 10–15 cases per 100,000 population. In 75% of patients, the hemorrhage occurs from a ruptured aneurysm, and in the remainder, it is caused by an arteriovenous malformation or bleeding disorder.

## PRESENTATION

Two-thirds of the patients are between the ages of 40 and 60 years. Women are affected slightly more frequently than men, possibly because of the higher prevalence of hypertension in women. Sometimes the hemorrhage is precipitated by an activity such as lifting, straining, intercourse, or emotional excitement. However, it can also occur during sleep, probably related to the increase in blood pressure during rapid eye movement sleep.

## DIAGNOSIS

Headache of hyperacute onset is the characteristic presentation of subarachnoid hemorrhage. The rapid onset of the headache is *the* key to diagnosis. The patient should be asked explicitly how fast the headache developed: seconds? minutes? hours? The headache of subarachnoid hemorrhage develops in a matter of seconds, like a blow to the head or neck. If this is the history, the diagnostic process should be pursued to the point of lumbar puncture. The lumbar puncture should, however, *always* be preceded by neurodiagnostic imaging (computed tomography without contrast), if available, and should be performed when the imaging is negative.

On examination, the key finding in subarachnoid hemorrhage is limited forward flexion of the neck with intact rotation. The limitation in forward flexion is due to chemical inflammation of the meninges, and this sign takes several hours to develop. Preretinal hemorrhages, seen on examination of the fundi, occur in large hemorrhages only.

The ultimate diagnostic test in subarachnoid hemorrhage is lumbar puncture and spinal fluid analysis. If the patient is *not* seriously ill, it is important to wait 6 hours after the onset of headache before performing the lumbar puncture. This makes it easier to distinguish a positive result from a traumatic tap when the cerebrospinal fluid is hemorrhagic. Centrifugation of the spinal fluid yields yellow fluid in the case of hemorrhage and colorless fluid in a traumatic tap.

# Hypertensive Encephalopathy

A 34-year-old woman is in the fifth month of her second pregnancy. She has been feeling very tired and has had a severe headache for almost a week. The headache is located in the back of the head and is somewhat worse on the right side. It is throbbing in nature and is associated with nausea but not with vomiting. On examination, the blood pressure is 160 over 110 mm Hg, with a pulse rate of 84 beats per minute. There is slight pitting edema of the ankles. The fundi are unremarkable. Blood chemistry reveals an elevated blood urea nitrogen of 25 mg per dl and an elevated thyroid-stimulating hormone level of 5.9 µU per ml. Quantitative urinalysis shows an increase in creatinine clearance to 188 ml per minute. She is treated with metoprolol (Lopressor) and levothyroxine (Synthroid), which rapidly improve the blood pressure and relieve the headache.

## PATHOGENESIS

Hypertensive encephalopathy occurs when blood pressure increases acutely beyond the level of cerebral autoregulation. The autoregulation failure allows the increase in blood pressure to be transmitted to the cerebral circulation, ultimately resulting in cerebral edema. Headache is often an early symptom and develops even before the cerebral edema occurs. In this early stage, the headache is due to distention of the cerebral arteries at the base of the skull, where they are sensitive to pain. Once cerebral edema has developed, the headache is caused by traction on the bridging veins to the superior sagittal sinus.

## PRESENTATION

Apart from headache, there may be blurring of vision, mental changes, or even seizures. Papilledema is generally also present at this point as a result of the increased intracranial pressure. The blood pressure necessary to cause hypertensive encephalopathy depends on the usual blood pressure of the patient. If the blood pressure is low, a moderate elevation (e.g., 150/90) may suffice. If the blood pressure is chronically elevated, however, a very high blood pressure (e.g., 220/130) may be required. This makes it difficult to evaluate the situation solely on an absolute reading of the blood pressure.

## ETIOLOGY

Hypertensive encephalopathy occurs in chronically hypertensive patients as well as in patients with normal blood pressure. In hypertensive patients, it tends to occur when blood pressure is poorly controlled, and it may be precipitated by heavy salt intake. In otherwise normotensive patients, the acute increase in blood pressure may be caused by toxemia of pregnancy, as in the patient described in the previous case study, or by acute glomerulonephritis. Hypertensive encephalopathy can also occur when a patient on a monoamine oxidase inhibitor for the treatment of depression ingests tyramine-containing food or uses a decongestant.

## DIAGNOSIS

The headache of hypertensive encephalopathy is generalized in location and usually more frontal than occipital. The headache may be associated with nausea when more intense. Blurring of vision is also common, and flashing or shimmering lights (photopsia) may be associated with it.

Funduscopy may reveal the arteriolar changes of chronic hypertension. It may also show the papilledema, exudates, and hemorrhages of severe uncontrolled hypertension. In the previously healthy and normotensive patient, the fundi may be unremarkable or may show signs of arteriolar constriction. Computed tomography may show hypodense areas, especially in the so-called *watershed zones* between the territories of the major cerebral arteries. On lumbar puncture, the pressure as well as the protein content of the spinal fluid may be elevated.

# Treatment of Acute Headache

Parenterally administered medications are generally used to treat headache in the emergency room. Table 6-1 lists the medications that have been studied in the treatment of acute, severe headache in the emergency room. They are ranked according to their efficacy in decreasing headache intensity within 1 hour of administration.

## CHOICE OF MEDICATIONS

Prochlorperazine (Compazine), given slowly and intravenously in a dose of 10 mg, seems most effective, with an efficacy of 88% in providing complete or partial pain relief.[1] Second in effectiveness is

**Table 6-1. Efficacy of medications in the treatment of acute, severe headache**

| Medication | Efficacy (%) |
|---|---|
| Prochlorperazine, 10 mg IV[a] | 88 |
| Chlorpromazine, 12.5–37.5 mg IV[b] | 80 |
| Dihydroergotamine, 1 mg IV with metoclopramide, 10 mg IV[c] | 70 |
| Metoclopramide, 10 mg IV[d] | 67 |
| Butorphanol, 2 mg IM[c] | 64 |
| Ketorolac, 60 mg IM[e] | 55 |
| Lidocaine, 50–150 mg IV[b] | 50 |
| Meperidine, 75 mg IM with hydroxyzine, 50 mg IM[c] | 45 |
| Dihydroergotamine, 1–2 mg IV[b] | 37 |

IV = intravenously; IM = intramuscularly.
[a]J Jones, D Sklar, J Dougherty, et al. Randomized double-blind trial of intravenous prochlorperazine for the treatment of acute headache. JAMA 1989;261:1174–1176.
[b]R Bell, D Montoya, A Shuaib, et al. A comparative trial of three agents in the treatment of acute migraine headache. Ann Emerg Med 1990;19:1079–1082.
[c]MJ Belgrade, LJ Ling, MB Schleevogt, et al. Comparison of single-dose meperidine, butorphanol, and dihydroergotamine in the treatment of vascular headache. Neurology 1989;39:590–592.
[d]DS Tek, DS McClellan, JS Olshaker, et al. A prospective, double-blind study of metoclopramide hydrochloride for the control of migraine in the emergency department. Ann Emerg Med 1990;19:1083–1087.
[e]RN Harden, TD Carter, CS Gilman, et al. Ketorolac in acute headache management. Headache 1991;31:463–464.

chlorpromazine (Thorazine), also given intravenously, which has an efficacy of 80%.[2] In the comparative trial by Bell et al.,[2] the chlorpromazine was given in intravenous boluses of 12.5 mg, and, if necessary, repeated twice at intervals of 20 minutes, with a maximum of 37.5 mg. Before administration of the medication, the patients were given 500 ml normal saline intravenously. This may have decreased the occurrence of hypotension often seen with intravenous administration of chlorpromazine, an effect that is much less common with prochlorperazine. Other side effects of either prochlorperazine or chlorpromazine, both phenothiazines, are sedation and dystonia.

Next in line in efficacy is metoclopramide (Reglan), either alone or in combination with dihydroergotamine (D.H.E. 45). Metoclopramide, when given in a dose of 10 mg intravenously, has an efficacy of 67% in providing effective pain relief.[3] Adding dihydroergotamine in a dose of 1 mg intravenously increases metoclopramide's efficacy in relieving headache to 70%.[4] Dihydroergotamine alone, on the other hand, in a dose of 1–2 mg intravenously has an efficacy of only 37%.[2] Dihydroergotamine should *never* be given without prior administration of an antinausea medication. When it is given alone, the resulting nausea or vomiting may negate any beneficial effect on the headache.

Of the opioid medications studied, only butorphanol (Stadol) has a relatively good efficacy (64%).[4] The combination of meperidine (Demerol) and hydroxyzine (Vistaril) has an efficacy of only

45%.[4] Nevertheless, this combination is still the treatment of acute, severe headache most commonly employed in emergency rooms.

Ketorolac (Toradol), the nonsteroidal anti-inflammatory analgesic available for parenteral administration, has a somewhat better efficacy of 55%.[5] However, my own experience with this medication has been rather disappointing. More effective is the specific antimigraine medication, sumatriptan (Imitrex). In a dose of 6 mg subcutaneously, its efficacy is 70% in decreasing the intensity of moderate or severe headache to mild or no headache.[6]

Dihydroergotamine and sumatriptan are potent arterial vasoconstrictors and therefore should not be used in patients with uncontrolled hypertension or coronary artery disease.

## PERSONAL APPROACH

### First Step

My own approach to the treatment of acute, severe headache is to start by giving the patient 10 mg metoclopramide intramuscularly or intravenously (Table 6-2). Metoclopramide is a very effective antinausea medication without contraindications

**Table 6-2. A three-step approach to the treatment of acute, severe headache**

1. Metoclopramide, 10 mg IM or IV, followed by
2. Diazepam, 5–10 mg IV when muscular symptoms (neck tightness) are prominent, followed by
3. Dihydroergotamine, 0.5 mg IM, repeated if necessary after 30 mins

IV = intravenously; IM = intramuscularly.

and with few side effects. It does not have cardio-vascular effects and therefore can be safely given as an intravenous bolus. Sometimes it causes restless-ness (akathisia) as a side effect and, rarely, dystonia. The dystonia usually occurs in adolescent or young adult women and generally involves stiffness of the tongue. This can be reversed easily with diphenhy-dramine (Benadryl), administered in a dose of 50–100 mg intravenously.

Metoclopramide does not cause drowsiness and therefore can be given to the patient with acute, severe headache before the diagnostic process is ini-tiated. As a result of its severe intensity, acute head-ache is often associated with nausea or vomiting. Metoclopramide effectively relieves the gastroin-testinal symptoms and makes it easier for the patient *and* physician to go through the diagnostic process.

## Second Step

Once the diagnostic process is complete and treatment can be continued, I give 5–10 mg diazepam (Valium) intravenously when muscular symptoms, such as tightness of the neck muscles, are prominent.

## Third Step

Otherwise, or with any remaining headache, I give dihydroergotamine, 0.5 mg intramuscularly, which I repeat, if necessary, after 30 minutes. In my experience, giving the dihydroergotamine intravenously does not provide better relief than the intramuscular route. On the other hand, gastrointestinal and possibly cardiac[7] side effects occur more often with intravenous than with intramuscular administration of the medication.

The advantage of dihydroergotamine over sumatriptan is dihydroergotamine's longer duration of action, which, in my experience, has been associated with less recurrence of headache. Headache recurrence can be further decreased by adding a corticosteroid to the treatment, for example, dexamethasone (Decadron) 4–8 mg intravenously.

# REFERENCES

1. Jones J, Sklar D, Dougherty J, White W. Randomized double-blind trial of intravenous prochlorperazine for the treatment of acute headache. JAMA 1989;261:1174–1176.
2. Bell R, Montoya D, Shuaib A, Lee MA. A comparative trial of three agents in the treatment of acute migraine headache. Ann Emerg Med 1990;19:1079–1082.
3. Tek DS, McClellan DS, Olshaker JS, et al. A prospective, double-blind study of metoclopramide hydrochloride for the control of migraine in the emergency department. Ann Emerg Med 1990;19:1083–1087.
4. Belgrade MJ, Ling LJ, Schleevogt MB, et al. Comparison of single-dose meperidine, butorphanol, and dihydroergotamine in the treatment of vascular headache. Neurology 1989;39:590–592.
5. Harden RN, Carter TD, Gilman CS, et al. Ketorolac in acute headache management. Headache 1991;31:463–464.
6. Cady RK, Wendt JK, Kirchner JR, et al. Treatment of acute migraine with subcutaneous sumatriptan. JAMA 1991;265:2831–2835.
7. Galer BS, Lipton RB, Solomon S, et al. Myocardial ischemia related to ergot alkaloids: a case report and literature review. Headache 1991;31:446–450.

# PART TWO

# Subacute Headache

# Clinical Approach to Subacute Headache

Subacute headache is defined as a headache that has been present for days or weeks, as opposed to acute headache, which has been present for hours or days. Cerebral tumor, pseudotumor cerebri, ophthalmic zoster, temporal arteritis, and subdural hematoma are possible causes of subacute headache.

## CEREBRAL TUMOR IN CHILDHOOD

Cerebral tumor is especially a concern in children. In adults, cerebral tumors are usually located in a cerebral hemisphere and therefore give rise to neurologic symptoms or signs early in the course of illness. In children, however, they are often located in the posterior fossa. There, they easily obstruct the flow of cerebrospinal fluid, causing headache *without* neurologic symptoms.

The most common cerebral tumors in childhood are medulloblastoma (a malignant tumor of the cerebellar vermis), ependymoma (a tumor of the fourth ventricle), cerebellar astrocytoma (a malignant tumor of the cerebellar hemisphere), and pontine glioma (a malignant tumor of the pons). In children, certain details in the history should raise suspicion of a cerebral tumor as the cause of headache, including[1]

1. Headache on awakening in the morning
2. Being awakened by headache at night
3. Persistence of headache at high intensity
4. Changing nature or frequency of headache

From the general history, a change in behavior or school performance, or both, can be added to this list.

## NEUROLOGIC EVALUATION OF THE CHILD WITH HEADACHE

In the evaluation of headache in childhood, the neurologic examination is very important and should include an evaluation of the visual acuity and fundi.[1] In children with headache due to cerebral tumor, 55% show abnormalities on the examination within 2 weeks of headache onset. Within 2 months, 85% show abnormalities, and after 6 months, *all* children with headache due to cerebral tumor have abnormalities on the neurologic examination.

## REFERENCE

1. Honig PJ, Charney EB. Children with brain tumor headache. Am J Dis Child 1982;136:121–124.

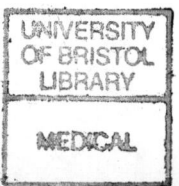

# Cerebral Tumor

A 37-year-old woman complains of persistent headaches in the right temple. The headaches started 2–3 weeks before consultation. They are mild in intensity but present continuously. Initially, the headaches were nothing more than a throbbing sensation. They are not associated with any other symptoms, and nothing in particular preceded their onset. Nonprescription analgesics provide temporary relief, but the patient takes them only sporadically. She had breast cancer several years earlier, which was treated with mastectomy and radiation. On examination, she shows slight drooping of the left corner of her mouth and clumsiness of the left hand. Computed tomography with contrast reveals a round lesion in the right parietal lobe, surrounded by extensive edema, as is typical of a metastatic tumor (Fig. 8-1).

## ETIOLOGY

Cerebral tumors are divided into primary and secondary (metastatic). Metastatic tumors account for 30% of all intracranial tumors. They reach the brain through hematogenic seeding, most notoriously from lung or breast cancer. Much less common sources of metastatic cerebral tumors are hypernephroma and melanoma. By the time the cerebral metastasis occurs, the primary tumor is generally known. A cerebral metastasis may be the first manifestation of the illness, however, particularly with lung cancer.

## INCIDENCE

The incidence of primary cerebral tumors in the United States is estimated at 5–10 cases per 100,000 population per year. Those affected are mostly between the ages of 50 and 70 years. In half the cases, the tumor originates from the glial cells of the brain and is a glioma. In 60% of patients with

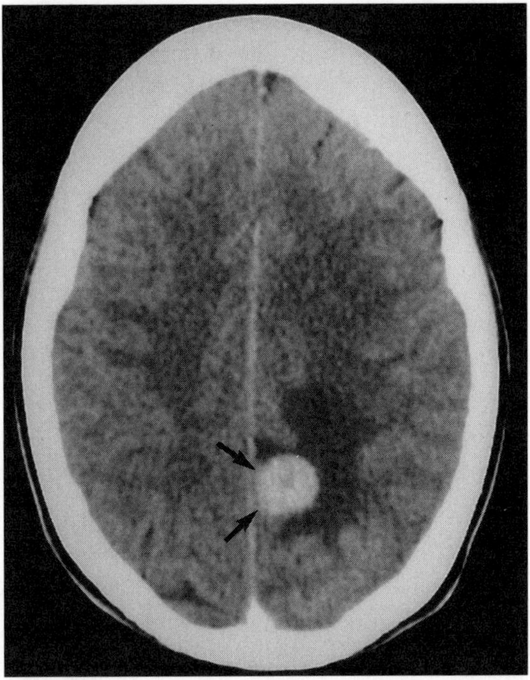

**Figure 8-1.** Computed tomogram with contrast shows a metastasis of breast cancer in the right parietal lobe (arrows), surrounded by edema.

glioma, the glioma is a so-called *malignant glioma* or *glioma multiforme*. This is a very malignant tumor with a short duration of illness, often leading to death within 6 months to 1 year.

---

## GLIOMA

---

A 30-year-old woman is brought to the emergency room because of a generalized seizure associated with urinary incontinence. The seizure left her drowsy and with a severe, generalized, throbbing headache. The neurologic examination was otherwise unremarkable. An electroencephalogram showed focal slowing over the left anterior region. Magnetic resonance imaging revealed a low-grade glioma in the left frontal lobe (Fig. 8-2). A craniotomy was performed with gross total resection of the tumor. Pathologic examination determined the tumor to be a grade II/IV astrocytoma. The resection was followed by external beam radiation.

---

The initial manifestation of a malignant glioma is generally not headache but neurologic symptoms or seizure. A seizure without obvious cause in

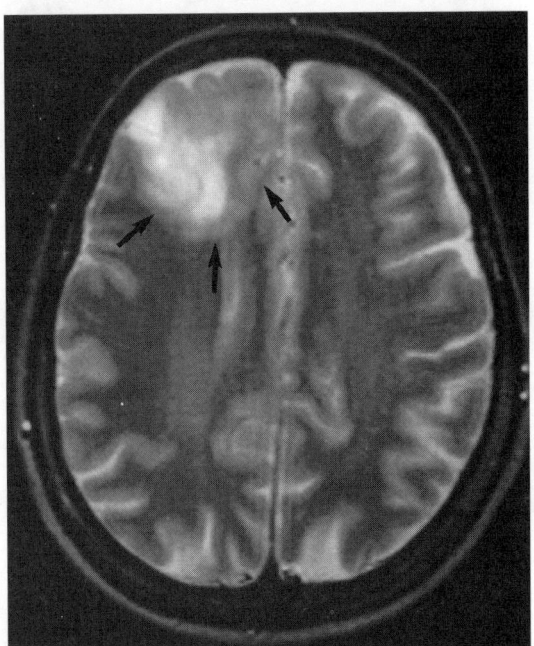

**Figure 8-2.** Magnetic resonance imaging shows a low-grade glioma in the left frontal lobe (arrows). (Courtesy of Patrick Y. Wen, M.D., Boston, MA.)

adulthood should *always* be considered a symptom of cerebral pathology until proved otherwise.

The other gliomas, astrocytoma and oligodendroglioma, have a much less disastrous course than malignant glioma but are still malignant. They grow slowly but invasively, generally leading to death within 3–5 years. They generally also present with neurologic symptoms or seizure, but the symptoms progress very slowly and can be very subtle. Abnormalities on neurologic examination may be found early in the course of illness if the examination is performed meticulously and, if necessary, repeated.

## MENINGIOMA

The cerebral tumor that occurs almost as frequently as glioma is meningioma, a benign tumor that originates from the dura mater. It occurs three times more frequently in women than in men. It is often located over a cerebral hemisphere and manifests itself through headache or seizure. Nonfocal neurologic symptoms, such as lack of perseverance, emotional lability, and memory impairment, generally occur before local symptoms develop. The nonfocal neurologic symptoms are due to edema of cerebral tissue adjacent to the tumor. Although it is discussed under Subacute Headache, the headache caused by meningioma is often chronic because it is a very slow-growing tumor. The following case study illustrates this.

---

A 33-year-old woman has had headaches for 7 years. As a result of a gradual increase in frequency, the headaches have occurred daily for the last year. Over time, the headaches have also become some-what more intense and longer-lasting. They now generally start around noon and last for the remain-der of the day. The headaches were initially mild but have become moderate in intensity and less responsive to nonprescription analgesics. They are not associated with nausea, vomiting, photophobia, or phonophobia but are accompanied by some soreness of the neck and shoulder muscles. The headaches are located on the right in the forehead but, when more intense, become bifrontal. Approxi-mately a year before consultation, she experienced a feeling of pins-and-needles in the left side of her body that lasted a week. On examination, her reflexes are brisker on the left than on the right, with a pathologic plantar response on the left; the optic disks are normal. Computed tomography with con-trast shows a lesion located high frontoparietally on the right (Fig. 8-3). Angiography confirms that the lesion is a meningioma.

---

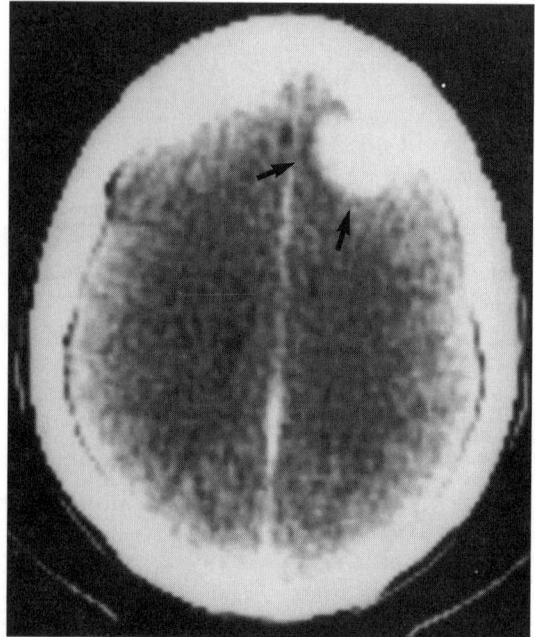

**Figure 8-3.** Computed tomogram with contrast shows a meningioma on the right in the frontoparietal area (arrows).

The headache caused by a meningioma is localized to the side of the tumor but is not necessarily limited to its exact location. It may be intermittent or continuous, and it usually progresses in intensity over time. Gastrointestinal symptoms, if associated with the headache, are generally not very prominent. The headache may be easily mistaken for a tension-type headache or migraine. The localization of the headache *always* on the same side (fixed lateralization) as well as its gradual progression should raise suspicion. The preferential diagnostic test for meningioma is neurodiagnostic imaging. Computed tomography shows the tumor as a hyperdense lesion, which further increases in density after administration of contrast.

## OTHER SYMPTOMS AND SIGNS

When a cerebral tumor reaches a certain size, causes edema, or obstructs the flow of cerebrospinal fluid, increased intracranial pressure results. At this point, generalized headache develops, independent of the location of the tumor. Vomiting, typically explosive and with minimal or no associated nausea, may also occur, as well as a decrease in the level of consciousness. On neurologic examination, the increased intracranial pressure is evident from the presence of papilledema, at least in the younger patient.

# Pseudotumor Cerebri

A 50-year-old woman presents with generalized
weakness and headaches. The weakness started
2–3 months before consultation and the headaches 1
month before. The headaches have been daily and
continuous since their onset. Initially, they were mild in
intensity and were relieved by nonprescription analgesics. The headaches gradually became more
intense and have been severe for the last week, waking her out of sleep every night. They are present on
awakening in the morning and fluctuate in intensity
over the day but not in any particular pattern. The
headaches are located in the back of the neck and
extend from there into the back and top of the head,
temples, and eyes. They are sharp and steady in

nature. They are associated with tingling on top of the head and, at times, with pressure in the ears. The headaches are also associated with anorexia, photophobia, phonophobia, and blurring of vision. Physical activity, coughing, and bending over make the headaches worse, but applying a hot towel around the head makes them somewhat better. She has had Crohn's disease for 4 years, which has rendered her anemic, with a hemoglobin of 9.8 g per dl; her sedimentation rate is 79 mm per hour. On examination, the margins of her optic disks are blurred, and venous pulsations are absent. Computed tomography is normal, and a lumbar puncture reveals the spinal fluid pressure to be elevated at 230 mm $H_2O$.

## SYMPTOMS AND SIGNS

Pseudotumor cerebri is a condition of increased intracranial pressure caused by impaired absorption of cerebrospinal fluid or edematous swelling of the brain, or both. It occurs most often in patients younger than age 40 years and is two or three times more common in women than in men.

Headache is present in more than 80% of patients and is generalized in location. It tends to be dull and steady in nature but may become worse with sudden movements of the head, coughing,

**Table 9-1. Common symptoms of pseudotumor cerebri**

Headache
Blurring of vision
Double vision (on lateral gaze)
Visual obscuration

sneezing, straining, or bending over. It is usually not associated with nausea but may be associated with vomiting, especially on rising in the morning.

Blurring of vision and double vision are other symptoms often encountered (Table 9-1). The blurring of vision may relate to the papilledema, which is the most significant finding in the condition, although it is occasionally absent. Other possible findings on ophthalmologic examination are decreased visual acuity and visual field defects, especially enlargement of the blind spots and a restriction of peripheral vision.

The double vision relates to impaired function of one or both abducens (i.e., sixth cranial) nerves due to compression. Double vision occurs on lateral gaze and is a nonspecific symptom of increased intracranial pressure.

A symptom that may be more characteristic of pseudotumor cerebri is a transient loss of vision on getting up quickly from lying down or sitting. It sometimes also occurs with coughing, sneezing, straining, or bending over. It lasts seconds and is similar to the loss of vision experienced presyncopally but is not associated with feeling faint.

## ETIOLOGY

Pseudotumor cerebri is associated with morbid obesity, and this may account for as much as half of the cases. Obesity is associated with increased central venous pressure, which causes an increase in intracranial venous pressure. This, in turn, impairs the absorption of cerebrospinal fluid (through the arachnoid villi) into the superior sagittal sinus.

An increase in intracranial venous pressure can also be caused by venous obstruction from, for example, venous sinus thrombosis. Venous sinus thrombosis can occur during pregnancy or oral contraceptive use, two scenarios that have also been causally related to pseudotumor cerebri. Other possible causes of the condition are excessive vitamin A intake, abrupt corticosteroid withdrawal, severe anemia, and hypothyroidism.

## DIAGNOSIS

The diagnosis of pseudotumor cerebri is made through lumbar puncture, which often reveals a markedly elevated pressure, generally in the range of 300–400 mm $H_2O$. The lumbar puncture should *always* be performed after neurodiagnostic imaging to rule out a space-occupying lesion and biventricular or triventricular hydrocephalus. In pseudotumor cerebri, neurodiagnostic imaging typically shows slitlike ventricles, which are indicative of diffuse cerebral edema. In addition, the sella may appear empty, which, like papilledema and abducens paresis, is another consequence of increased intracranial pressure (empty sella syndrome).

## TREATMENT

The treatment of pseudotumor cerebri consists of repeated lumbar punctures to decrease the intracranial pressure. The repeated lumbar punctures alone sometimes "cure" the condition. If this is not effective, a lumboperitoneal shunt may be considered for effective drainage of the spinal fluid. Some suggest treatment with a high dose of a corticosteroid before placing a lumboperitoneal drain. Acetazolamide (Diamox), a carbonic anhydrase inhibitor, can also be given to decrease the formation of cerebrospinal fluid. In cases involving severe papilledema, optic nerve sheath fenestration may be indicated to spare vision.

# Ophthalmic Zoster

A 69-year-old woman complains of excruciating headaches in the left forehead and anterior vertex. The headaches started 1–2 weeks before consultation and have been present continuously since. They are steady and so intense that they prevent her from doing anything during the day. In the evening, the headaches make it very difficult for her to fall asleep, and at night, they wake her up. The area involved in the headaches is very sensitive to touch and, when touched, the pain feels like sharp knives. On examination, the left upper eyelid is found to be very red and swollen and has a little round lesion on it, covered by a crust. She is referred to an ophthalmologist for further examination of the eye.

## HERPES ZOSTER

Ophthalmic zoster is a form of herpes zoster with symptoms and signs in the distribution of the ophthalmic nerve. The ophthalmic nerve is the division of the trigeminal nerve that innervates the forehead and anterior vertex. Herpes zoster is caused by the varicella-zoster virus, which is the same virus that causes chickenpox. After chickenpox, the virus resides in the sensory ganglia, particularly the trigeminal and thoracic. It remains latent in the ganglia until it is reactivated by waning immunity. As a result, the incidence of herpes zoster increases progressively with advancing age.

During chickenpox, the virus migrates from the cutaneous vesicles along the sensory nerve fibers to the ganglia. Once reactivated in a ganglion, it causes necrotic inflammation of the ganglion and moves along the nerve fibers back to the skin. In the skin, it multiplies in the epidermal layer, leading to the formation of vesicles.

## OPHTHALMIC ZOSTER

By age 85 years, half of the population has had herpes zoster, and ophthalmic zoster accounts for 10–15% of all cases. The sexes are equally affected, as are the sides of the body.

With ophthalmic zoster, the pathologic changes occur in the trigeminal ganglion. The ipsilateral forehead or anterior vertex, or both, usually feel very sensitive several days before the vesicular eruption. The sensitivity may be associated with a burning or tingling sensation, particularly when the skin is touched. However, there can also be pain, at times severe, and the diagnosis is generally not clear until the vesicles appear. The vesicles occur in clusters, and the skin is generally red and swollen. They are initially clear but are later cloudy, and they become dry and crusty within 1–2 weeks. The sensitivity and the pain, if present, abate in most cases within 1–4 weeks but may persist for months or years (postherpetic neuralgia). On examination, decreased sensation can often be found in the affected dermatome for weeks or months after the acute episode.

## TREATMENT

The main hazard of ophthalmic zoster is involvement of the cornea, leading to scarring of the cornea and decreased vision. Prolonged pain, so-called *postherpetic neuralgia*, is also a feared but rare sequel of the condition.

Treatment of the acute episode consists of acyclovir (Zovirax) 800 mg five times per day for 7 days. When treatment is started within 48 hours of appearance of the vesicles, the vesicles heal more quickly and the pain associated with them lasts for a shorter amount of time. In addition, the patient can also be given acyclovir applied topically to the eye, either as a solution or as an ointment.

# Temporal Arteritis

A 76-year-old man is brought to the office by his wife. Over the weeks preceding the consultation, he has become increasingly irritable and confused. He started behaving as if he had lost his senses. He also does not want to eat anymore. During the day, his wife cannot get him out of his chair, and at night he does not want to sleep. She tried to keep him in bed for a couple of days, but to no avail. His only complaint is headache, which he describes as a sharp pain in the head. Nonprescription analgesics give him only slight relief. The only thing that helps are warm compresses applied to the head. On examination, he looks sweaty and is disoriented in time. His temperature is 100.2°F (37.9°C). His neck is difficult to move in any direction. The blood pressure is 145 over 70 mm Hg, with a pulse rate of 92 beats per minute. His temporal arteries are prominently visible, possibly due to thickening, but they pulsate normally. On laboratory testing, the white blood cell count is 8,600 cells per µl, and the sedimentation rate is 96 mm per hour. The temporal artery biopsy is positive for temporal arteritis (Fig. 11-1). On prednisone, 80 mg per day, his senses return within days, and the headache vanishes.

## ETIOLOGY

Temporal arteritis is a condition that affects the elastic arteries, with a preference for those of the head (cranial arteritis). Anatomically, it is characterized by necrosis of the media, which, in elastic arteries, is predominantly made up of elastin. The necrosis is associated with the formation of granulomatous tissue and giant cells (giant cell arteritis). The cause of the condition is unknown but probably involves the generation of autoantibodies against elastin.

## PRESENTATION

Temporal arteritis occurs almost exclusively after age 60 years and affects men and women equally. It is a

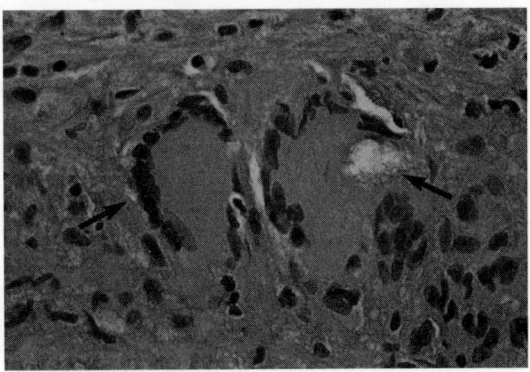

**Figure 11-1.** Biopsy of the temporal artery shows two multinuclear giant cells (arrows) characteristic of temporal arteritis.

relatively rare condition whose incidence increases with age.

## SPECIFIC AND SYSTEMIC SYMPTOMS

The symptoms can be divided into those specific for the arteries involved and those reflecting the systemic, inflammatory nature of the condition (Table 11-1). The systemic symptoms include general malaise, generalized weakness, easy fatigability, lack of appetite, weight loss, and low-grade fever.

**Table 11-1. Specific and systemic symptoms of temporal arteritis**

| Category | Symptoms |
|----------|----------|
| Specific | Headache |
|          | Jaw "claudication" |
|          | Blindness |
|          | Stroke |
| Systemic | General malaise |
|          | Generalized weakness |
|          | Easy fatigability |
|          | Lack of appetite |
|          | Weight loss |
|          | Low-grade fever |

The low-grade fever can often be detected only by having the patient measure his or her temperature several times per day.

Headache is probably the most common specific symptom of temporal arteritis due to the preference of the condition for the arteries of the head, particularly the temporal arteries. The headache is often severe and is described as a deep, burning pain, sometimes with a throbbing quality. It is caused by dilation of the larger extracranial arteries, the lumina of which are narrowed by swelling of the vessel wall. In addition, the vessel wall is very sensitive to stretch due to the inflammatory process affecting the arteries. Ischemia of the scalp is another factor contributing to the headache of temporal arteritis. The ischemia explains why heat applied to the head often diminishes the intensity of the pain.

Another specific symptom of temporal arteritis that originates from the extracranial circulation is "claudication" of the muscles of mastication. The patient complains of pain in the jaw muscles on prolonged chewing due to ischemia of the muscles. This symptom is often considered pathognomonic of the condition. Temporal arteritis sometimes affects the cerebral arteries, resulting in encephalopathy, with symptoms of apathy, confusion, and disorientation. When the cerebral arteries are involved, ischemic stroke may occur, with focal neurologic symptoms, such as aphasia, hemiparesis, or hemianopia.

## EXAMINATION

On physical examination, specific abnormalities are generally not found. A low-grade fever may be present but is easily missed because of its fluctuating course. The temporal arteries may be more clearly visible or more pronounced on palpation but characteristically show absent or diminished pulsations.

Routine laboratory testing typically reveals a strongly elevated sedimentation rate, slight anemia, and a slightly elevated alkaline phosphatase. The sedimentation rate is generally increased to 50–100 mm per hour but may also be normal. This means that in case of strong clinical suspicion, even with a normal sedimentation rate, a biopsy of the temporal artery should *always* be performed. For the biopsy, a reasonably long segment of the temporal artery should be excised. This is important because the lesions may not be present along the entire course of the blood vessel.

## TREATMENT

In 30% of cases, temporal arteritis also affects the ophthalmic arteries, leading to partial or total blindness due to retinal ischemia. It is because of this potential complication that the condition, once suspected, should be treated immediately while awaiting the biopsy.

Treatment consists of corticosteroids, which generally have a positive effect on the course of the illness. Otherwise, the condition is self-limiting, and the symptoms gradually disappear over the course of several months. Nonsteroidal anti-inflammatory analgesics are often effective in relieving the symptoms of temporal arteritis, such as headache, but they do not reduce the potential risk of blindness.

# Subdural Hematoma

A 72-year-old man is brought to the office by his wife because of headaches, drowsiness, and confusion. The headaches started 6 days before consultation and built slowly in intensity. They are located across the forehead and are not associated with any other symptoms. He does not have fever, and nothing in particular preceded the onset of the headaches. The drowsiness and confusion began 3 days after the headaches did. There is no recent history of head trauma, but his wife remarks that he often hits his head against the cabinet hanging over the work-bench. He has had two heart attacks and has since been on warfarin (Coumadin). His prothrombin time is 19.1 seconds. Computed tomography reveals

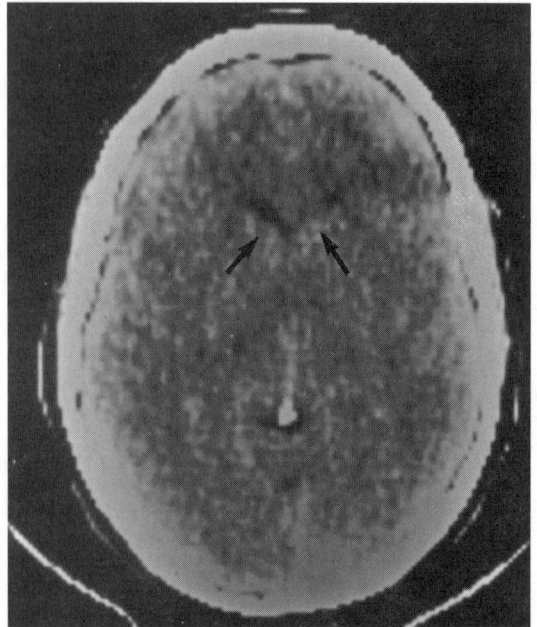

**Figure 12-1.** Computed tomogram shows "hypernormal" ventricles (arrows) and absent peripheral sulci.

"hypernormal" ventricles—that is, ventricles that are too small for his age—and absent peripheral sulci (Fig. 12-1). Angiography shows that the abnormal findings on computed tomography are due to bilat-

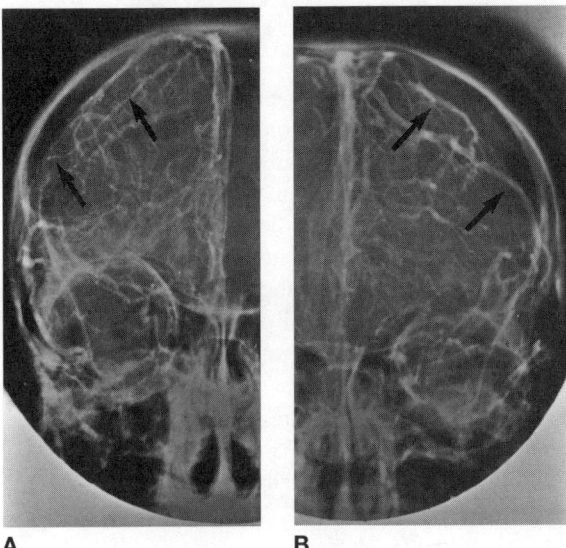

A          B

**Figure 12-2.** Angiogram shows displacement of blood vessels away from the skull on the left (A) and right (B) (arrows), consistent with bilateral subdural hematoma (same patient as in Fig. 12-1).

eral subdural hematoma (Fig. 12-2). Warfarin is discontinued, and he is treated with vitamin K. His mental status gradually improves, and so do the headaches.

## ETIOLOGY

Subdural hematoma is *always* the result of a head injury. In the elderly, however, the injury may be minimal and easily forgotten. Also, confusion and impairment of memory are common symptoms of the condition, which makes it difficult to obtain an accurate history. Subdural hematoma is a hematoma of venous origin located between the dura mater and arachnoid. It is generally located over the cerebral hemisphere and can be unilateral or bilateral. The cause of the hematoma is rupture of a bridging vein resulting from trauma to the head. However, it is almost never associated with fracture of the skull, indicating the generally mild nature of the head injury.

## PRESENTATION

Apart from infants, subdural hematoma predominantly occurs in patients older than age 50 years, and its incidence, such as that of ophthalmic zoster and temporal arteritis, increases with age. The relationship of the condition with age is connected to the brain's progressive shrinkage over the years. As a result, the bridging veins of the brain become more and more stretched, rendering them progressively more susceptible to injury. The use of antico-agulants as well as alcohol abuse further contribute to the risk of occurrence of subdural hematoma.

## SYMPTOMS AND SIGNS

Subdural hematoma is more common in men than in women. Headache is most frequently its present-ing symptom, but it may be absent. Headache is generally mild in intensity, present continuously, and localized to the side of the hematoma. Often, no other symptoms are associated with it. Mental symptoms, particularly confusion, disorientation, and drowsiness, are also common presenting symp-toms. Focal neurologic symptoms or signs, such as hemiparesis and asymmetric or pathologic reflexes, are much less common. Also, papilledema is hardly ever seen with subdural hematoma because it pre-dominantly affects the elderly. In the elderly, papilledema generally does not occur with space-occupying intracranial lesions because of the large replaceable cerebrospinal fluid volume.

## DIAGNOSIS

Subdural hematoma is diagnosed with neurodiag-nostic imaging. Depending on the age of the hematoma, computed tomography shows it as hyper-dense, isodense, or hypodense. When isodense, the only manifestation of the hematoma may be a shift of midline structures without further abnormalities. Magnetic resonance imaging or angiography may then be necessary to establish the presence of the hematoma.

## TREATMENT

Subdural hematoma can be treated either medically or surgically. Medical treatment consists of corticosteroids, which may be preferable to surgical treatment in the very old patient. Surgical treatment consists of evacuation of the hematoma and is associated with the general risks of surgery. Another problem with this surgery in the very old patient is that the brain may not expand after evacuation of the hematoma, resulting in a subdural space filled with air. Generally, patients improve with either treatment, but the improvement may be slow and only partial.

# PART THREE

# Chronic Headache

# CHAPTER THIRTEEN

# Clinical Approach to Chronic Headache

## PRESENTATION

In patients with chronic headache, the headaches have been present, either intermittently or continuously, for months or years and sometimes even decades. The patient with chronic headache is generally between 20 and 50 years of age because these are the years of highest headache prevalence. The patient is also more likely to be a woman than a man because headaches in women are more intense than those in men, resulting in a higher likelihood that women will seek medical care. Men and women have headaches equally frequently, but headaches of moderate and severe intensity are twice as common in women as in men.

---

## **ETIOLOGY**

---

Analysis of a database of more than 1,000 patients with chronic headache who sought specialty care for their headaches revealed that 75% of them were women and 25% men.[1] Their mean and median age at the time of consultation was 40 years. In almost half of the patients, the onset of their headaches occurred before age 20 years. In one-third of these patients, onset occurred in childhood (age 9 years or younger), in one-third in the early teens (age 10–14 years), and in one-third in the late teens (age 15–19 years). Of the patients with pre–adult-onset headache, almost 10% related the onset of their headaches to a specific circumstance, excluding menarche. In the patients with onset of headaches at age 20 years or older (adult-onset headache), this was the case in almost 40%. Table 13-1 lists the five most common circumstances of headache onset mentioned by the patients with adult-onset chronic headache.

In a separate (questionnaire) study of almost 200 patients with chronic headache, 20% related the onset of their headaches to the onset of menstruation.[2] When only the women were considered, the onset of headache was related to menarche by

**Table 13-1. Circumstances of headache onset in patients with adult-onset chronic headache (n = 221)**

| Circumstance | Percentage of patients |
|---|---|
| Head, neck, or back injury | 29 |
| Stress (illness, death, marriage, move, school, wedding, work) | 17 |
| Illness or surgery | 14 |
| Pregnancy (during or after) | 12 |
| Estrogen therapy (birth control, menopause) | 9 |

Source: Adapted from KM Karpouzis, ELH Spierings. Circumstances of onset of chronic headache in patients attending a specialty practice. Submitted for publication, 1998.

almost 30% of patients. In the study, half of the patients experienced headaches daily.

## DAILY HEADACHES

Daily headaches have been shown to affect 6% of the population 20 years of age and older: 4% of men and 8% of women.[3] It has the highest prevalence in the age groups of 20–24 years (8%) and older than 64 years (8%) and the lowest in the age group of 35–54 years (5%).

Daily headaches can be divided into paroxysmal and nonparoxysmal.

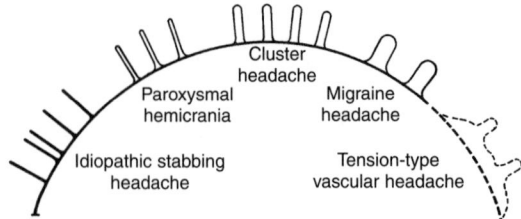

**Figure 13-1.** The spectrum of vascular headaches includes idiopathic stabbing headache, paroxysmal hemicrania, cluster headache, and migraine headache. (Drawn by Richard J. MacCormack, Sandwich, MA.)

## Paroxysmal

The paroxysmal daily headaches include cluster headache (see Chapter 22), paroxysmal hemicrania (see Chapter 24), and idiopathic stabbing headache (see Chapter 25). Together with migraine, these paroxysmal daily headaches constitute what I have referred to as the *spectrum of vascular headaches* (Fig. 13-1). They account for only a small fraction of the total daily headaches, however.

## Nonparoxysmal

The vast majority of daily headaches are nonparoxysmal (i.e., they lack a well-defined headache attack pattern) and are referred to as *chronic daily headache* (see Chapter 21).

## CRANIOCERVICAL MUSCLE TIGHTNESS

Chronic headache generally relates to an abnormal functioning of extracranial tissues, particularly muscles and arteries. Patients with chronic headache have increased tightness of the neck and jaw muscles, as was demonstrated in a study that looked at 164 headache patients and compared them with 108 age- and gender-matched controls (Table 13-2).[4] The patients had had headaches for an average of 14 years. Tightness of the neck muscles was reported by 49% of the headache patients compared to 30% of the controls. The

**Table 13-2. Muscle tightness in patients with chronic headache versus age- and gender-matched controls**

|  | Tight neck muscles (% of patients) | Tight jaw muscles (% of patients) |
|---|---|---|
| Controls (n = 108) | 30 | 17 |
| Headache patients (n = 164) | | |
|     While headache-free | 49 | 17 |
|     During headache | 69 | 30 |

Source: Adapted from J Lebbink, ELH Spierings, HB Messinger. A questionnaire survey of muscular symptoms in chronic headache. Clin J Pain 1991;7:95–101.

prevalence of neck-muscle tightness in the headache patients increased to 69% when headache was actually present. Tightness of the jaw muscles was equally common in the headache patients and the controls (17%), but its prevalence was increased in the headache patients when headache was present (30%). The tight jaw muscles during headache may be the result of the increased tightness of the neck muscles. It has been shown in animal experiments that noxious stimulation of neck muscles increases the electromyographic activity of jaw muscles, but stimulation of jaw muscles does not increase the activity of neck muscles.

## CRANIOCERVICAL ELECTROMYOGRAPHIC ACTIVITY

Similar observations as in the muscle-tightness study were made in an electromyographic study of 19 headache patients and 12 controls.[5] The electromyographic activity of the neck muscles was higher in the headache patients than in the controls. No differences were found between the patients with muscle-contraction headache and those with migraine, whether headache was present or not. The lack of a significant difference in neck-muscle electromyographic activity during and between headaches, however, may have been due to the relatively small number of patients in the study compared to the muscle-tightness study. The same may be true for the negative finding with regard to the difference between muscle-contraction headache and migraine, which was not examined in the muscle-tightness study.

## MUSCULAR MECHANISM

It is known from other studies, however, that when it comes to electromyographic activity of cranio-cervical muscles, migraine patients tend to have higher activity than those with muscle-contraction or tension-type headache. This does not mean that muscle contraction is not an important mechanism in tension-type headache: It may mean that it is an even more important mechanism in migraine. In my experience, muscle contraction is often present when migraine headaches occur frequently and the patient is en route to developing chronic daily headache (see Chapter 14).

## VASCULAR MECHANISM

With regard to arterial involvement in headache, vasodilation causes pain by stretching of the nerve fibers that coil around the blood vessels. This mecha-

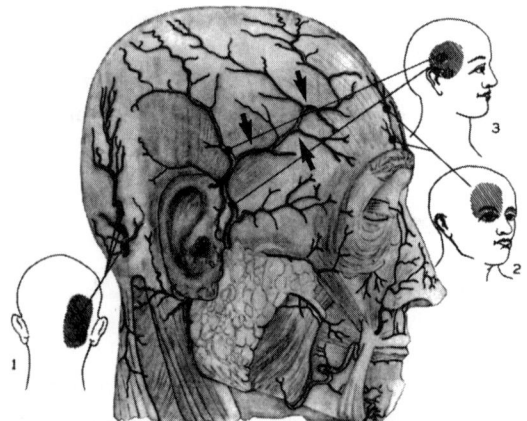

**Figure 13-2.** Superficial temporal artery (3), of which the frontal branch (arrows) is preferentially involved in the mechanism of migrainous vasodilation. (1 = occipital artery; 2 = supraorbital artery.) (Reprinted with permission from DJ Dalessio. Wolff's Headache and Other Head Pain. New York: Oxford University Press, 1972;214.)

nism has been implicated in migraine and cluster headache. It particularly involves the frontal branch of the superficial temporal artery (Fig. 13-2), giving rise to the throbbing pain in the temple so characteristic of migraine. Another prominent location of the headache that involves a vascular mechanism is in or behind the eye. This is typically the location of the headache in cluster headache, which is generally considered a migraine-related condition. Cluster headache is a chronic headache condition with a well-defined presentation and treatment (see Chapters 22 and 23).

## CLASSIFICATION

Much less well defined in their presentation than cluster headache are the two most common chronic headache conditions: tension-type headache and migraine. The distinction drawn between the two is relatively arbitrary, despite the fact that the International Headache Society has published strict criteria for the diagnosis of the two conditions.[6] These criteria, which are summarized in Table 13-3, are overlapping, lack biological validity, and have not been tested clinically.[7] They should therefore only be used as guidelines in the diagnostic process, if used at all.

### Table 13-3. International Headache Society's diagnostic criteria for migraine and tension-type headache

Migraine (code 1.1)
  A. At least five attacks fulfilling conditions B–D, below
  B. Attacks lasting 4–72 hrs
  C. Headache has at least two of the following characteristics:
    1. Unilateral location
    2. Pulsating quality
    3. Moderate or severe intensity
    4. Aggravated by routine physical activity
  D. During headache, at least one of the following:
    1. Nausea or vomiting
    2. Photophobia and phonophobia
Tension-type headache (code 2.1)
  A. At least 10 episodes fulfilling criteria B–D, below
  B. Episodes last from 30 mins to 7 days
  C. Headache has at least two of the following characteristics:
    1. Pressing or tightening quality
    2. Mild or moderate intensity
    3. Bilateral location
    4. Not aggravated by routine physical activity
  D. During headache, both of the following:
    1. No nausea or vomiting
    2. Photophobia or phonophobia

Source: Adapted from International Headache Society. Classification and diagnostic criteria for headache disorders, cranial neuralgias and facial pain. Cephalalgia 1988;8(suppl 7):1–96.

# REFERENCES

1. Karpouzis KM, Spierings ELH. Circumstances of onset of chronic headache in patients attending a specialty practice. Submitted for publication, 1998.
2. Spierings ELH. Onset and relief of headache in patients attending a headache practice: a survey. Headache Q 1996;4:324–325.
3. Instituut Epidemiologie. Epidemiologisch Preventief Onderzoek Zoetermeer (EPOZ): Tweede en Derde Voortgangsverslag. Rotterdam, The Netherlands: Erasmus University, 1976.
4. Lebbink J, Spierings ELH, Messinger HB. A questionnaire survey of muscular symptoms in chronic headache. Clin J Pain 1991;7:95–101.
5. Pritchard DW. EMG cranial muscle levels in headache sufferers before and during headache. Headache 1989;29:103–108.
6. International Headache Society. Classification and diagnostic criteria for headache disorders, cranial neuralgias and facial pain. Cephalalgia 1988;8 (suppl 7):1–96.
7. Messinger HB, Spierings ELH, Vincent AJP. Overlap of migraine and tension-type headache in the International Headache Society classification. Cephalalgia 1991;11:233–237.

# CHAPTER FOURTEEN

# Headache Continuum

Clinically, tension-type headache and migraine fall on a continuum (Fig. 14-1). It is referred to as a *continuum* because of the many intermediary stages that exist between the headache syndromes: migraine, episodic and chronic tension-type headache, and tension-type vascular headache. This differs from the spectrum of vascular headaches discussed in Chapter 13, in which intermediary stages are rare or nonexistent.

The episodic form of tension-type headache stands at one end of the continuum and migraine at the other end. In between are chronic tension-type headache and tension-type vascular headache. In the classification of the International Headache Society, tension-type vascular headache is referred to as *migraine with chronic tension-type headache.*

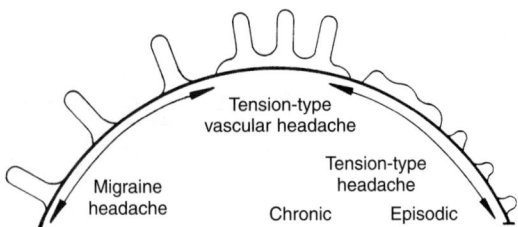

**Figure 14-1.** The continuum of headache syndromes includes episodic and chronic tension-type headache, tension-type vascular headache, and migraine headache. (Drawn by Richard J. MacCormack, Sandwich, MA.)

Most of these patients have one rather than two headache conditions, however, and a single diagnosis is therefore more appropriate. The following two case studies illustrate the difference between migraine with chronic tension-type headache and tension-type vascular headache.

---

A 46-year-old woman has had headaches since her teens. Initially, the headaches occurred twice per week, began in the late afternoon, and were relieved by non-prescription analgesics. They were mild in intensity and not associated with any other symptoms. The headaches gradually increased in frequency and became daily when she was approximately 20 years old. They also started earlier in the day and are now present on awakening 2 days per week. Otherwise, the headaches begin in the early afternoon. They are mild to moderate in intensity and still respond to nonprescription analgesics. The headaches are located like a band across the forehead and are associated with tenderness of the suboccipitalis and temporalis muscles. The neck and shoulder muscles are tight. Since her mid-20s, the patient has also experienced severe headaches that do not respond to nonprescription analgesics. They occur once per month but are not related to menstrual periods. The severe headaches are brought on by not eating on time, exposure to sun, and sometimes alcohol. They begin during the day, build to their maximum intensity in 2–3 hours, and last 24 hours. The headaches are located in the right eye and are sharp and steady in nature. They are associated with nausea, vomiting, photophobia, and phonophobia as well as with blurring of vision, especially in the right eye. Noise, light, physical activity, and bending over make the headaches worse, but lying down makes them somewhat better.

A 53-year-old woman has had headaches since early childhood. Initially, the headaches were severe in intensity and associated with nausea and vomiting. They gradually increased in frequency but became somewhat less intense and less associated with vomiting. In her teens, the headaches occurred once or twice per week. They occurred even more frequently when she was in her early 20s but were not yet daily. The headaches have been daily for the last 10–20 years. They are present on awakening in the morning and are worst at that time. The headaches wake her out of sleep in the early morning two or three times per week. The severe headaches occur once or twice per week and last 1–3 days. The headaches are located on one side or the other, with a preference for the right, in the eye, temple, and side of the head. They are usually dull and steady but are sometimes throbbing. The headaches are associated with photophobia and phonophobia and, when severe, with nausea. They are also associated with very tight and sore neck and shoulder muscles, worse on the right. The jaw muscles are also very tight but not sore. Fluorescent light, stress, fatigue, hunger, and physical activity make the headaches worse. Before menopause, they were also worse premenstrually. Lying down makes the headaches somewhat better, as does applying heat to and massaging the back of the neck and forehead.

## ANALYSIS OF CASES

The first patient started with episodic tension-type headache in her teens and gradually progressed to chronic tension-type headache at approximately age 20 years. In her mid-20s, a migraine condition developed independent of the chronic tension-type headache, with well-defined headaches distinct from the daily headaches. The second patient had severe migraine headaches from early childhood on. The headaches gradually increased in frequency to daily occurrence, with the migraine headaches immersed in the daily headaches. This condition could also be referred to as *chronic migraine*, if that term were in use. The prominence of muscular symptoms in association with the migraine headaches has led to the designation of combined vascular and muscle-contraction headache.[1] I prefer the term *muscle-contraction vascular headache* and have translated that into *tension-type vascular headache* to conform with the terminology used by the International Headache Society. The second case is not that of migraine with chronic tension-type headache because, clearly, only one headache condition has developed, over time, out of migraine.

## HEADACHE DYNAMICS

Patients with tension-type headache or migraine can present anywhere on the continuum and can, in the course of time, move along it, as indicated by the arrows in Fig. 14-1 and as illustrated by the two case studies. The sole basis for the continuum is the clinical presentation of the headaches, with the many intermediary stages between tension-type headache and migraine. The continuum speaks to the frustration a physician often feels in trying to decide whether a patient has tension-type headache or migraine, especially when the headaches occur frequently. It does not imply that tension-type headache and migraine are caused by the same mechanism, however.

## HEADACHE MECHANISMS

### A Common Mechanism

A common mechanism for tension-type headache and migraine has been suggested, among others, by my mentor in headache, John R. Graham. In the 1930s, Dr. Graham and Harold G. Wolff established the vascular mechanism of migraine—namely, that the migraine headache is caused, at least in part, by dilation of extracranial arteries.[2] Through clinical headache work spanning half a century, Dr. Graham came to believe that *all* chronic headaches are vascular, including muscle-contraction headache, which is now called *tension-type headache.*

## Interaction of Mechanisms

In my opinion, the physiologic basis of the headache continuum lies in the interaction between the muscular and vascular mechanisms of headache. In this interaction, the vascular mechanism, through the intense pain it generates, activates the muscular mechanism. The activation of the muscular mechanism consists of involuntary contraction of the craniocervical muscles. The muscular mechanism, in turn, activates the vascular mechanism through mechanical interference with muscle circulation. The decreased circulation causes the body to respond with dilation of the feeding arteries, such as the frontal branch of the superficial temporal artery (see Chapter 13, Fig. 13-2), which overlies the powerful temporalis muscle.

## MECHANISM IN RELATION TO HEADACHE INTENSITY

### Muscular Mechanism

The muscular mechanism by itself generates headaches of mild to moderate intensity, diffuse location, and pressing quality (Table 14-1). The

**Table 14-1. Presentation of headache, depending on the mechanism involved**

| Mechanism | Headache characteristics |
|-----------|--------------------------|
| Muscular | Mild to moderate intensity |
| | Diffuse location |
| | Pressing quality |
| | Develops during the day |
| | Lacks associated symptoms |
| Vascular | Moderate to severe intensity |
| | Localized to the temple or eye |
| | Throbbing quality |
| | Present on awakening |
| | With associated symptoms |

headaches usually develop during the day, often in the afternoon, and gradually build in intensity as the day progresses. They usually lack associated symptoms, such as photophobia or nausea, because of the relatively low intensity of the pain.

## Vascular Mechanism

The vascular mechanism, on the other hand, generates headaches of moderate to severe intensity. These headaches are often localized, usually to the temple or behind the eye, or both, and they are throbbing. They are often associated with other symptoms, such as photophobia, phonophobia, nausea, and vomiting. The headaches tend to be present on awakening in the morning or wake the patient out of sleep at night.

## REFERENCES

1. Ad Hoc Committee on Classification of Headache. Classification of headache. JAMA 1962;179:717–718.
2. Graham JR, Wolff HG. Mechanism of migraine headache and action of ergotamine tartrate. Arch Neurol Psychiatry 1938;39:737–763.

# Tension-Type Headache

A 35-year-old woman has had headaches for 2–3 years, dating from the time when she had her first child. The headaches occur once or twice per week and are brought on by lack of sleep. They usually begin in the early afternoon, when she starts to feel tired. The headaches are mild in intensity and are located across the forehead. They are not associated with any other symptoms. The headaches last for 1–2 hours and are relieved by nonprescription analgesics or rest. Her neck, shoulder, and jaw muscles are not tight or sore. She has two children, who are now 3 and 1½ years old. The children still regularly wake her up at night, and then she has difficulty going back to sleep.

## EPISODIC TENSION-TYPE HEADACHE

Tension-type headache can be episodic or chronic, depending on the frequency of occurrence of the headaches. The patient described in the preceding case study has episodic tension-type headache, with the headaches occurring once or twice per week.

The headaches in episodic tension-type headache are often thought to be brought on exclusively by stress or tension. This is not true, however, and fatigue, lack of sleep, and not eating on time are common triggers as well. The headaches usually begin during the day, typically in the late afternoon, and may be relieved by the evening. They are mild to moderate in intensity and generally not associated with any other symptoms, except for occasional mild photophobia or phonophobia. They tend to have a rather diffuse location (i.e., across the forehead, on top of, or in the back of the head), although they can be unilateral. The headaches generally respond well to nonprescription analgesics.

## CHRONIC TENSION-TYPE HEADACHE

In chronic tension-type headache, the headaches occur daily or almost daily. They are otherwise the same as in episodic tension-type headache, except that they are present on awakening in the morning or begin shortly after rising. The following case study is a typical presentation of chronic tension-type headache.

---

A 36-year-old woman has had headaches since her teens. The headaches have been daily since their onset. They are present on awakening in the morning and become somewhat more intense as the day progresses. The headaches are worst in the late afternoon but remain relatively mild. They are located bilaterally in the back of the head as a dull ache. The headaches are not associated with any other symptoms. Nothing in particular, including menstrual periods, makes them worse or better. Her neck and shoulder muscles are somewhat tight and sore.

---

## Etiology

Chronic tension-type headache can be caused by chronic anxiety, but this is rare in my experience. It is much more common for the condition to be related to chronic fatigue, often due to lack of sleep. The lack of sleep can be caused by problems falling asleep or sleeping through the night, but it can also be the result of a particular lifestyle. Some people believe that they should be able to function perfectly well with only 5–6 hours of sleep per night. Although a rare individual can do this, most people need at least 7–8 hours to function well. Whatever the cause, however, it is generally evident from the context in which the chronic tension-type headache presents, as the following case study illustrates.

---

A 32-year-old man has had headaches daily since his teens. The headaches are mild in intensity and located in the back of the head. They are associated with tightness of the neck and shoulder muscles. He has had anxiety since childhood. The anxiety is present daily and has gradually gotten worse over time. It is associated with worrying, difficulty concentrating, shortness of breath, sweating, and diarrhea. The anxiety is much more bothersome to him than the headaches, which he lists among the symptoms resulting from it.

---

Chronic tension-type headache is more often secondary than primary—that is, it generally develops out of episodic tension-type headache. This is not true in the two patients just described, whose headaches have been daily since their onset. When the chronic tension-type headache is primary, there is often a precipitating physical event, such as a whiplash injury of the neck or a flulike illness.

Sometimes, the event is meningitis, subarachnoid hemorrhage, or myelography, with the meningeal irritation initiating the contraction of the cranio-cervical muscles.

## Frequent Analgesic Use

The most common cause of episodic tension-type headache turning into chronic tension-type headache is treatment that relies on analgesics. Analgesics, whether nonprescription or prescription, address only the symptom of headache and neglect the underlying mechanism, resulting in a gradual increase in frequency of the headaches.

Frequent use of analgesics for headache also affects the efficacy of preventive treatment—that is, treatment aimed at decreasing the frequency, intensity, and duration of the headaches. Lee Kudrow was the first to demonstrate this in an elegant study of the effect of amitriptyline (Elavil) on chronic muscle-contraction headache.[1] He showed that the medication was less than half as effective (30% versus 72%) in patients who were allowed to take analgesics for their headaches compared to those who were not. This negative effect of frequent analgesic use for headache is not limited to amitriptyline, however; it extends to all pharmacologic and nonpharmacologic preventive treatments for headache. Therefore, with frequently occurring headaches, even when these headaches are mild, it is important to obtain accurate information about the intake of both prescription and nonprescription analgesics. The information should include the number of tablets taken per day and the number of days per week or per month that the medications are taken. When analgesics are taken more often than 1–2 days per week, they must be discontinued as the first step of treatment.

Discontinuation of analgesic use is often followed by an improvement of the headaches, even without the prescription of preventive treatment. The analgesics are generally best discontinued abruptly rather than tapered. Abrupt discontinuation is often followed by an initial worsening of the headaches for 2–3 days. Patients must be informed of this so that they know what to expect. Patients can be prescribed muscle relaxants, such as metaxalone (Skelaxin) or carisoprodol (Soma), as needed for their headaches.

## REFERENCE

1. Kudrow L. Paradoxical effects of frequent analgesic use. Adv Neurol 1982;33:335–341.

# Treatment of Tension-Type Headache

## PHARMACOLOGIC TREATMENT

The two medications that have been shown to be effective in the preventive treatment of chronic tension headache are amitriptyline (Elavil)[1,2] and doxepin (Sinequan)[3] (Table 16-1). These agents are best prescribed once daily at bedtime because they often cause sedation. The dosages used for the treatment of headache (25–75 mg per day) are lower than those for depression. Apart from sedation, the medications can cause dry mouth, constipation, and weight gain. They are particularly helpful in patients who also have problems falling asleep or sleeping through the night.

**Table 16-1. Medications effective in the preventive treatment of tension-type headache**

| Medications | Dose | Side effects | Contraindications |
|---|---|---|---|
| Amitriptyline (Elavil) Doxepin (Sinequan) | 25–75 mg at bedtime | Sedation, dry mouth, constipation, weight gain | Glaucoma, prostate hypertrophy, epilepsy, cardiac arrhythmias |

I usually initiate treatment with a dose of 25 mg at bedtime and gradually increase the dose until some dryness of the mouth occurs. At the same time, I watch for the effect on the headaches and the occurrence of other side effects, particularly weight gain. Once the headaches are under control, I gradually decrease the dose to see whether the patient can do without the medication or to find the lowest effective dose.

Both amitriptyline and doxepin increase serotonin activity in the central nervous system. As a result, they inhibit central pain transmission and increase the pain threshold. The medications may also have a muscle-relaxant effect, possibly mediated by their anticholinergic activity.

In case the patient does not tolerate amitriptyline or doxepin because of excessive drowsiness or weight gain, another tricyclic can be tried. A tricyclic that I might use under these circumstances is imipramine (Tofranil). This medication has been shown to be effective in the treatment of chronic tension headache, but only in an open study.[4] Imipramine was less effective than amitriptyline, however, with 48% (imipramine) versus 74% (amitriptyline) of the patients responding with an improvement of 50% or more (placebo response: 33%).

Of the selective serotonin re-uptake inhibitors, paroxetine (Paxil) and fluvoxamine (Luvox) have been studied in the preventive treatment of chronic tension-type headache. Paroxetine was not effective,[5] whereas fluvoxamine, in a comparative study, significantly reduced the number of days with headache, headache intensity, and analgesic intake.[6]

## NONPHARMACOLOGIC TREATMENT

Aside from medications that relax the craniocervical muscles and prevent tension-type headache, treatment consists of physical therapy and relaxation therapy (Table 16-2).

### Physical Therapy

The simplest form of physical therapy is the use of a heating pad on the neck and shoulder muscles. This is often an effective way of decreasing the tightness of

**Table 16-2. Nonpharmacologic treatments of tension-type headache**

| Treatment | Modalities |
| --- | --- |
| Physical therapy | Daily use of a heating pad |
| | Stretching and strengthening exercises |
| | Massage, ultrasound, traction |
| | Myofascial release |
| | Mobilization and manipulation |
| Relaxation therapy | Autogenic training |
| | Biofeedback training |

neck and shoulder muscles, provided it is applied regularly, preferably daily. Exercises can be added to the use of the heating pad to stretch and strengthen the neck and shoulder muscles. More formal physical therapy modalities for these muscles include massage, ultrasound, traction, and myofascial release. Injection of the trapezius muscles with a local anesthetic, for example, can further help to relax the muscles. Mobilization or manipulation of the neck can also be helpful in stretching and thereby relaxing the small intervertebral muscles.

## Relaxation Therapy

Relaxation therapies that can be used are autogenic and biofeedback training. In autogenic training, suggestions of warmth and heaviness are used to relax successive parts of the body. Biofeedback training makes use of providing information to the patient about the state of contraction of the muscles. This generally makes it easier for the patient to learn to relax the muscles. The relaxation therapies, however, are only effective when practiced regularly, preferably daily. In this way, they do not differ from the preventive medications, which also must be taken daily to be effective.

## REFERENCES

1. Lance JW, Curran DA. Treatment of chronic tension headache. Lancet 1964;1:1236–1239.
2. Diamond S, Baltes BJ. Chronic tension headache treated with amitriptyline—a double-blind study. Headache 1971;11:110–116.
3. Morland TJ, Storli OV, Mogstad TE. Doxepin in the prophylactic treatment of mixed "vascular" and tension headache. Headache 1979;19:382–383.
4. Lance JW, Curran DA, Anthony M. Investigations into the mechanism and treatment of chronic headache. Med J Aust 1965;52:909–914.
5. Langemark M, Olesen J. Sulpiride and paroxetine in the treatment of chronic tension-type headache. An explanatory double-blind trial. Headache 1994;34:20–24.
6. Manna V, Bolino F, Di Cicco L. Chronic tension-type headache, mood depression and serotonin: therapeutic effects of fluvoxamine and mianserine. Headache 1994;34:44–49.

# Migraine

A 53-year-old woman has had headaches since age 13–14 years. Initially, the headaches occurred only with menstrual periods but not monthly. They were moderate in intensity and associated with nausea but not with vomiting. The headaches became more intense when she was in her early twenties and started taking oral contraceptives. Later, they occurred monthly, with periods, and lasted 1 day. When she was in her mid-40s, the headaches increased to every 2 weeks in frequency and to 2 days in duration. The headaches begin shortly after rising in the morning. Once every 2–6 weeks they wake her up at night. The headaches build to their maximum intensity in 2 hours. They are severe in intensity and associated with nausea, photophobia, and phonophobia. About half of the headaches are also associated with vomiting. They are located on one side of the head or the other, with a preference for the right, in the eye, and on top of the head. The headaches are steady and are made worse by light, noise, and physical activity. Lying down quietly in a dark room and applying ice to the back of the head and neck relieve the headaches somewhat. Food additives and preservatives bring on headache, as does rainy weather. Her neck, shoulder, and jaw muscles are tight and sore, especially on the right.

## PREVALENCE

The prevalence of migraine is 9% in men and 16% in women; it is 3–4% in children and is the same for boys and girls (Fig. 17-1).[1] Migraine is a condition of recurring headaches of moderate to severe intensity. The headaches generally last 1–3 days and occur at varying frequency. When occurring frequently (i.e., more than once or twice per month), they are often interspersed with tension-type headaches. The headache condition may gradually develop into tension-type vascular headache (see Chapter 14).

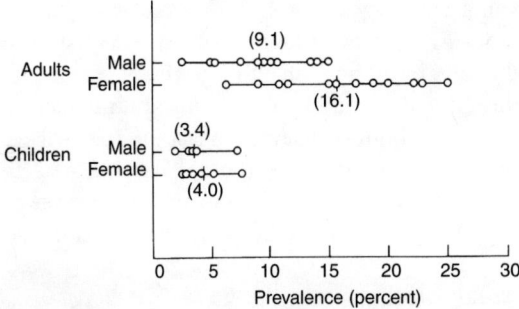

**Figure 17-1.** Prevalence of migraine in the general population, based on a review of epidemiologic studies. The numbers in parentheses are the means. (Reprinted with permission from M Goldstein, TC Chen. The epidemiology of disabling headache. Adv Neurol 1982;33:380.)

## MIGRAINE HEADACHE

The headaches of migraine tend to be limited to one side of the head and typically alternate sides. They are often located in the temple or the eye, or both, but they can also be in the back or on the top of the head. They are typically throbbing in the temple and in the back of the head but sharp and steady when located in the eye. Generally, the headaches are minimally associated with photophobia and phonophobia but often also with nausea and sometimes with vomiting. They are present on awakening in the morning, or they wake the patient out of sleep in the early morning. When they begin during the day, the headaches build to their maximum intensity over several hours. They often last for at least 1 day (e.g., they last until the end of the day and are gone by the next morning), but they can also continue for days. When a migraine headache lasts much longer than 3 days, it is referred to as *migraine status* or *status migrainosus*.

## MIGRAINE STATUS

The following case study illustrates migraine status.

A 51-year-old woman has had headaches for 15 years, starting after her last pregnancy. Initially, the headaches occurred once per month with menstrual periods and lasted 24–48 hours. They were severe but not associated with nausea or vomiting. When she was prescribed an oral contraceptive 4 years ago, the headaches became longer-lasting. They occurred during the placebo week and ultimately lasted for the full duration of that week. She discontinued the oral contraceptive 2 months ago and has had a severe headache since. It is a sharp, steady pain located in the left forehead, eye, and side of the nose. It is associated with phonophobia and photophobia, with the latter mostly in the left eye. The headache is made worse by light, noise, physical activity, bending over, reading, and watching television. Lying down quietly in a dark room and applying ice to the left side of the face give some relief. She takes prescription analgesics daily with some temporary benefit.

---

In this case, the migraine status was triggered by the discontinuation of the oral contraceptive and perpetuated by the daily intake of analgesics. Generally, it can be treated effectively by discontinuing analgesics, in combination with a short course of a corticosteroid. I usually prescribe prednisone (Deltasone) under the given circumstance for 3 days in a dosage of 60 mg the first day, 40 mg the second, and 20 mg the third.

## MIGRAINE TRIGGERS

### Menstrual Cycle

In women, as in the preceding two case studies, migraine headaches often occur in relation to the menstrual cycle—that is, with menstruation or ovulation, or both. When occurring perimenstrually,

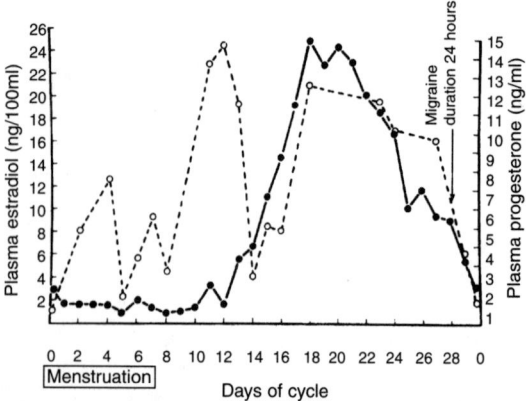

**Figure 17-2.** Plasma levels of estradiol (interrupted line) and progesterone (solid line) during the menstrual cycle in a woman with menstrual migraine. The arrow indicates the time of onset of the migraine attack. (Reprinted with permission from BW Somerville. The role of estradiol withdrawal in the etiology of menstrual migraine. Neurology 1972;22:357.)

the headaches tend to be particularly intense, incapacitating, and long lasting. Estrogens play an important role in menstrually related headaches, and their withdrawal has been shown to be related to the occurrence of migraine headache (Fig. 17-2).[2] The headaches tend to occur in relation to the menstrual cycle, especially when they start in the early teenage years or after pregnancy. Similarly, they are likely to occur with monthly bleeding when the patient is taking an oral contraceptive or is on cyclic menopausal estrogen therapy.

## Stress

Stress is also a common, although less potent, trigger of migraine. Typically, the headache comes after the stress—that is, when relaxation occurs. This is especially true when the headache develops during the evening or night after stress occurring in the preceding afternoon (Fig. 17-3).[3] The development of a migraine headache during the morning or afternoon has been related to tension occurring in the preceding days. When stress is added to the tension, fatigue results, which, if it is not relieved by a night's sleep, is followed by headache in the course of the morning (see Fig. 17-3). Otherwise, the tension changes into alertness, possibly due to relaxation of the body while the mind remains aroused. The next morning, the patient feels "stressed out," followed by extreme tension, irritability, and the development of headache in the course of the afternoon.

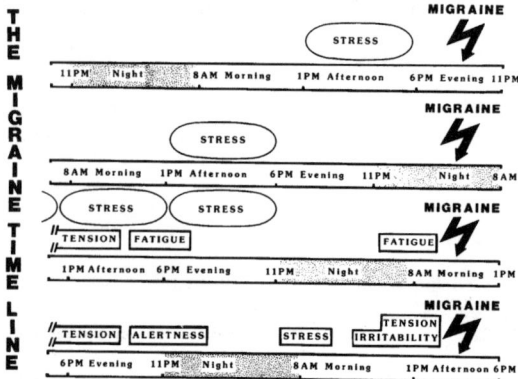

**Figure 17-3.** Psychophysical precedents of migraine in relation to the time of onset of the headache: the migraine time line. (Reprinted with permission from ELH Spierings, M Sorbi, GH Maassen, PC Honkoop. Psychophysical precedents of migraine in relation to the time of onset of the headache: the migraine time line. Headache 1997;37:219. Drawn by Richard J. MacCormack, Sandwich, MA.)

## Vasoactive Agents

Other important triggers of migraine are the vasoactive agents, which can be either vasodilators or vasoconstrictors (Table 17-1).

**Table 17-1. Vasoactive agents as triggers of migraine**

| Effect | Agent |
|---|---|
| Vasodilation | Alcohol |
| | Sodium nitrite (cured meat products) |
| Vasoconstriction | Caffeine |
| | Tyramine (cheese, red wine) |
| | Phenylethylamine (dark chocolate) |

### Vasodilators

Examples of vasodilator agents causing migraine are alcohol and sodium nitrite. Sodium nitrite is a food additive used to preserve meat and is present in cured meat products. The vasodilator agents precipitate a migraine headache through an indirect mechanism, which explains the delay in occurrence of the headache. The vasodilator effect of the agents causes peripheral vasodilation and a decrease in blood pressure, resulting in activation of the sympathetic nervous system that, in turn, is associated with vasoconstriction. The headache develops when the activation of the sympathetic nervous system wears off and cranial vasodilation occurs.

### Vasoconstrictors

Vasoconstrictor agents that cause migraine are caffeine and the sympathomimetic amines, tyramine and phenylethylamine. Caffeine causes headache on withdrawal (weekend migraine) when consumed in quantities of more than 200–300 mg per day, the equivalent of two or more cups of coffee.[4] Tyramine and phenylethylamine are chemicals present in dietary products, such as aged cheese, red wine, and dark chocolate. They act on the sympathetic nerve fibers and release from them the neurotransmitters noradrenaline and adrenaline. These neurotransmitters cause vasoconstriction, and the headache occurs as a result of the rebound vasodilation that follows the vasoconstriction.

## MIGRAINE MIMICS

Sometimes, other conditions masquerade as migraine; these conditions are referred to as *symptomatic migraine*. One such condition is chronic sinusitis, which can manifest as migraine without aura. Usually, although not always, nose and throat symptoms are present, such as nasal congestion and postnasal drip, which lead to the right diagnosis. However, patients may not mention these symptoms because they themselves do not see the connection with the headaches. Therefore, it is important in the evaluation of chronic headache to ask about persistent or recurring nose or throat symptoms. The following case study is that of a migraine-like condition caused by chronic sinusitis.

---

A 21-year-old man has had headaches for 2½ years. The headaches occur every 2–3 weeks when he exercises too much, especially when he has not had enough sleep. They are present on awakening the next morning and gradually improve over the next 2–3 days. The headaches are moderate in intensity and associated with anorexia and intermittently with nausea. They are centrally located in the head and sometimes also in the center of the face as a dull, steady pain. His nose has been congested since the onset of the headaches, somewhat worse on the right than on the left. Since that time, he has also had a severe postnasal drip with a bitter taste in the mouth and a foul breath. These symptoms become much worse after he exercises strenuously and before the onset of headache. Computed tomography of the sinuses reveals pansinusitis (Fig. 17-4).

---

Chronic sinusitis is best diagnosed with computed tomography, which must include coronal views of the nose and sinuses. Only then is it possible to evaluate the communications to the sinuses

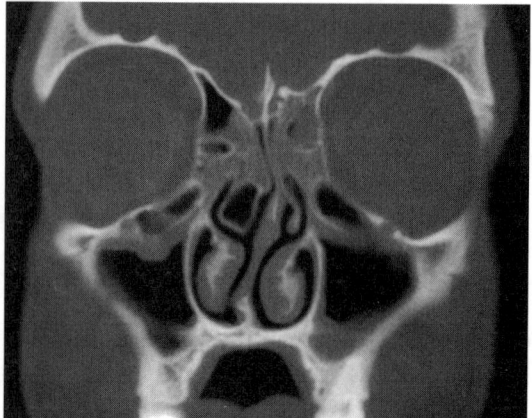

**Figure 17-4.** Computed tomogram of the sinuses shows extensive inflammation of the ethmoid sinuses and, to a lesser extent, of both maxillary sinuses.

(i.e., the ostiomeatal complexes and nasofrontal ducts). Medical treatment is generally most effective with an antibiotic that addresses anaerobic bacteria given in combination with a corticosteroid nasal spray. Sometimes, however, surgical treatment to open up the sinuses is unavoidable.

# REFERENCES

1. Goldstein M, Chen TC. The epidemiology of disabling headache. Adv Neurol 1982;33:377–390.
2. Somerville BW. The role of estradiol withdrawal in the etiology of menstrual migraine. Neurology 1972;22:355–365.
3. Spierings ELH, Sorbi M, Maassen GH, Honkoop PC. Psychophysical precedents of migraine in relation to the time of onset of the headache: the migraine time line. Headache 1997;37:217–220.
4. Shirlow MJ, Mathers CD. A study of caffeine consumption and symptoms: indigestion, palpitations, tremor, headache and insomnia. Int J Epidemiol 1985;14:239–248.

# CHAPTER EIGHTEEN

# Migraine Aura

A 27-year-old woman has had headaches since age 13 years, when she started menstruating. The headaches occur once per month perimenstrually and sometimes also with ovulation. They begin during the day, build to their maximum intensity in 30 minutes to 1 hour, and last for 1–2 days. The headaches are severe and are associated with nausea, irritability, photophobia, phonophobia, and osmophobia. They are located on the right behind the eye, in the temple, and in the back of the head. The headaches have a sharp, steady quality that gradually changes into a dull, throbbing pain. They are preceded by a visual disturbance that lasts for 15–20 minutes. The disturbance affects both visual fields but is more pronounced on the right. It consists of diagonal zigzag lines that move across the visual field from the bottom left to the top right. The zigzag lines are white-silver, look like lightning, and vibrate.

A 55-year-old man has had headaches since age 14 years. The headaches occur once per week and last for 1–2 days. They start in the course of the morning and build to their maximum intensity in 30 minutes. The headaches start on one side or the other in the frontotemporal area and become generalized from there. They are usually moderate in intensity and are associated with nausea, photophobia, phonophobia, and blurring of vision. The headaches are preceded by a visual disturbance, consisting of a distortion of vision, bright lights, and lightning patterns. The visual disturbance starts a half hour before the onset of the headache, in one visual field or the other, but always opposite to the side of the headache. After its onset and, like the headache, the visual disturbance becomes generalized to involve both visual fields. It lasts for 2–3 hours into the headache.

## VISUAL DISTURBANCE

The visual migraine aura has also been described in these ways:

- A blind spot gradually expanding into the left visual field and lasting for 30–45 minutes

- Tiny, silvery, and slightly colored crossmarks expanding from the center of vision into one peripheral field or the other, lasting for 20–25 minutes

- A sunburst in the left visual field, expanding into a circle surrounded by spikes, lasting for 20–25 minutes

- Colorful zigzag lines in one visual field or the other with a preference for the left, lasting for 30 minutes

- Prisms in the periphery of both visual fields, lasting for 20–30 minutes.

In classic migraine, or migraine with aura, the headaches are preceded by transient focal neurologic symptoms, generally known as *aura symptoms*. These aura symptoms are sensory in nature (either visual or somatosensory), although occasionally a speech disturbance occurs. The visual dis-

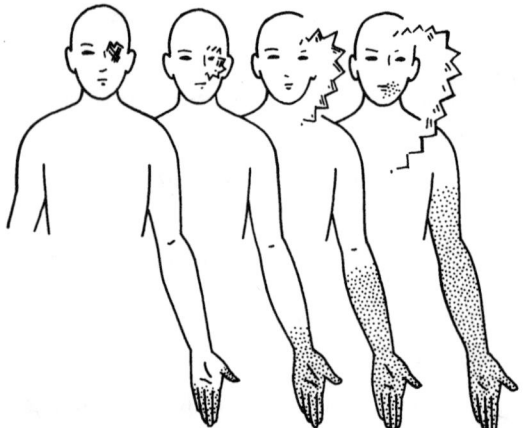

**Figure 18-1.** Scintillating scotoma (face area) and digitolingual paresthesias (hand, arm, and mouth area), shown from left to right in successive stages of development.

turbance typical of migraine is the scintillating scotoma, also called *teichopsia* or *fortification spectra* (Fig. 18-1). The scintillating scotoma usually starts near the center of vision as a small spot surrounded by bright, often flickering, and sometimes colorful zigzag lines. After slight enlargement, the circle of zigzag lines breaks open on the inside to take the form of a crescent, which gradually further expands into the periphery of a visual field. Vision is often obscured not only by the zigzag lines but also by a band of dimness that lies against it on the inside of the crescent.

From its onset near the center of vision to its disappearance in the periphery of a visual field, the scintillating scotoma lasts for 10–30 minutes, with an average of 20 minutes.

## SOMATOSENSORY DISTURBANCE

The somatosensory disturbance lasts for about the same length of time as the scintillating scotoma and it typically presents in the form of digitolingual paresthesias, also called *cheiro-oral syndrome* (see Fig. 18-1). These paresthesias consist of a feeling of tingling or pins-and-needles, and they start in the fingers of one hand. They gradually extend upward into the arm, ultimately to involve the face, especially the nose and mouth area, on the same side.

The somatosensory disturbance generally follows the visual disturbance but can also occur alone, although this is uncommon. The headache follows the visual or somatosensory disturbance either right away or after a certain interval (e.g., 1 hour). The headache is often unilateral in location and can be on the same side as the visual or somato-sensory disturbance or on the opposite side.

The next case study describes a patient with a somatosensory as well as a speech disturbance preceding the headaches.

---

A 37-year-old man has had headaches since age 5 years, but they have occurred more frequently since age 32 years. Presently the headaches occur five to six times per month and last 1–3 days. They are located bilaterally in the temples as a throbbing pain. The headaches are severe in intensity and are associated with nausea, vomiting, photophobia, and phonophobia. They are preceded by a sensation of pins-and-needles on one side of the body or the other, without preference. The pins-and-needles start in the fingers of one hand and gradually move up to involve the entire arm within 10 minutes. The arm and hand then feel weak, although the patient is able to move them. Once the pins-and-needles have reached the shoulder, they also occur around the mouth on the same side. He then experiences problems speaking, particularly in pronouncing words. The symptoms last for 10–30 minutes, depending on how far they progress.

---

## PATHOGENESIS

### Spreading Oligemia

The aura symptoms of migraine have long been thought to result from spasm of a cerebral artery, leading to localized and transient hypoxia of the brain. This notion is based on experiments in which it was shown that inhalation of a cerebral vasodilator, such as carbon dioxide or amyl nitrite, is followed by a temporary regression of the aura symptoms. However, cerebral blood flow studies have shown an initial *increase* in blood flow in the occipitoparietal area, followed by a *decrease* in blood flow and a gradual spreading of the decrease toward the frontal pole (Fig. 18-2).[1] The decrease is approximately 25%, which is not enough to cause neuronal dysfunction by ischemia and is therefore referred to as *oligemia* rather than *ischemia*.[2] The rate of forward spreading of the oligemia was determined to be 2.2 mm per minute.

### Spreading Depression

The particular nature of the cerebral blood flow changes has shed new light on a hypothesis that attributes the migraine aura to the neurophysiologic phenomenon of spreading depression.[3] Spreading

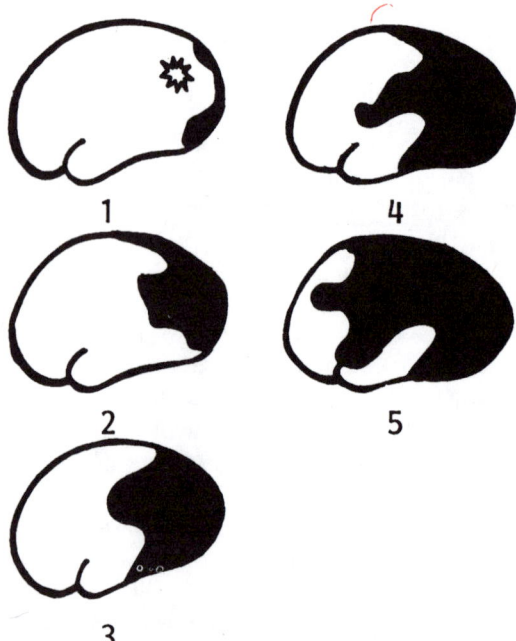

**Figure 18-2.** Changes in cerebral blood flow of the migraine aura in stages over time (1–5), described as *spreading oligemia*. The starburst indicates the initial increase in blood flow in the occipitoparietal area. The dark areas show the spreading oligemia. (Adapted from J Olesen, B Larsen, M Lauritzen. Focal hyperemia followed by spreading oligemia and impaired activation of rCBF in classic migraine. Ann Neurol 1981;9:344–352.)

depression is a wave of inhibition of neuronal activity that travels over the cerebral cortex at a rate of 2–5 mm per minute and is preceded by a brief phase of intense neuronal activity. The vascular changes accompanying spreading depression are similar to those that have been reported for the migraine aura: They consist of a brief increase in cerebral blood flow, followed by a longer-lasting decrease of 20–25%.[4]

## COMPLICATED MIGRAINE

Spasm of a cerebral artery is probably the mechanism related to complicated migraine, in which a stroke occurs during a migraine attack.[5] The stroke generally leaves a permanent neurologic deficit, such as a homonymous hemianopia or hemiparesis. The next case study is an example of migraine complicated by stroke, resulting in a permanent homonymous hemianopia.

A 30-year-old woman has had headaches since age 16 years, when she hit a tree while riding a motorcycle. The headaches occur seven to eight times per year and usually start in the late afternoon. They gradually build in intensity and are severe by the evening, forcing her to retire early. The headaches are almost always gone by the next morning. They are located across the forehead but then lateralize to the right temple with increasing intensity. The headaches are throbbing in the right temple. They are not associated with nausea, vomiting, photophobia, or phonophobia. One day she retired in the early evening because of a severe, throbbing headache in the right temple that had started in the afternoon. She became nauseated after she drank some lemonade and vomited all night. During the night, she noticed a pins-and-needles sensation in the left side of her body. In the early morning of the next day, she realized that she could not see well to the left with either eye. On examination, she had a homonymous hemianopia on the left, with sparing of central vision. Computed tomography showed decreased density in the territory of the right calcarine artery (Fig. 18-3). Vertebral angiography revealed irregular narrowing of the right posterior cerebral artery, suggesting vasospasm (Fig. 18-4).

## VARIANTS OF MIGRAINE WITH AURA

Two special forms of migraine that should be mentioned in the context of migraine with aura are

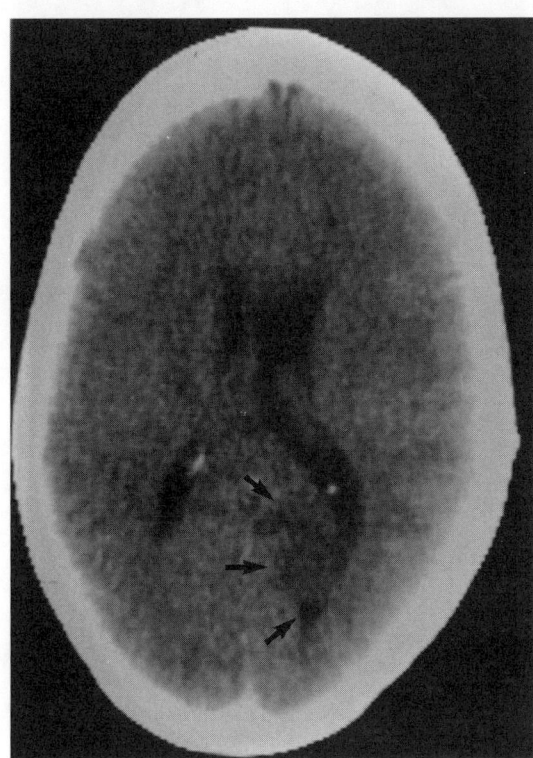

**Figure 18-3.** Computed tomogram shows an area of decreased density (infarct) in the territory of the right calcarine artery (arrows).

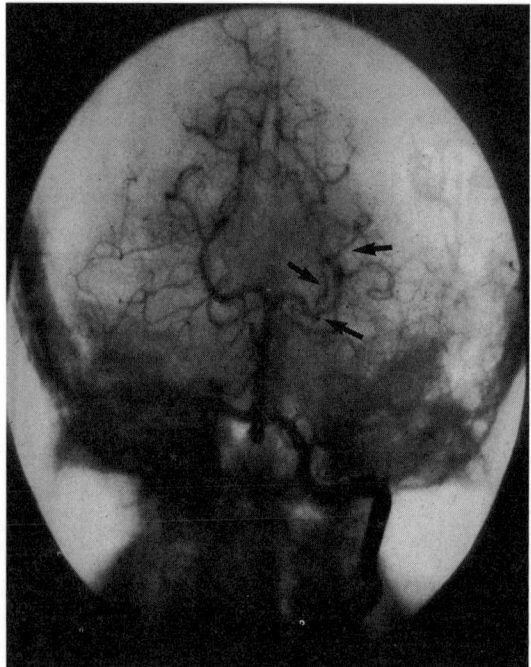

**Figure 18-4.** Vertebral angiogram shows irregular narrowing (vasospasm) of the right posterior cerebral artery (arrows). (Same patient as in Fig. 18-3.) (Reprinted with permission from ELH Spierings. Angiographic changes suggestive of vasospasm in migraine complicated by stroke. Headache 1990;30:728.)

hemiplegic and basilar migraine. They are considered variants of migraine with aura but are very rare.

## Hemiplegic Migraine

Hemiplegic migraine is best known in its familial form, which has been associated with genes on chromosomes 1 and 19. The following case study illustrates *non*familial hemiplegic migraine.

---

A 37-year-old woman has had headaches since age 10 years. The headaches occur two or three times per month and last for 2–3 days. They are present on awakening in the morning or begin during the day. The headaches build to their maximum intensity in 1 hour. They are severe in intensity and sharp and steady in nature. The headaches are located on one side or the other, with a preference for the right. They often start in the side of the nose and extend from there to behind the eye. Sometimes, the headaches start in the back of the neck. They are associated with photophobia and phonophobia as well as with throbbing of the temple on the side of the pain. When they start during the day, the headaches are preceded by a feeling of weakness in the arm and hand on the same side as where the pain later develops. The weakness is *not* associated with a feeling of tingling or pins-and-needles. It starts 1 hour before the onset of headache and lasts for the duration of the headaches.

---

## Basilar Migraine

In basilar migraine, the aura symptoms are thought to originate from the brain stem and include such symptoms as diplopia, bilateral paresthesias, and stupor. Basilar migraine needs to be differentiated from migraine associated with anxiety, hyperventilation, or vasovagal lability. The following case study illustrates basilar migraine.

---

A 22-year-old man has had headaches since age 9 years. The headaches occur once per month and last for 1–3 days. They start during the day and build to their maximum intensity in 1–2 hours. They are located bilaterally in the temples and in the sides of the head but are usually worse on the right. They are severe, sharp, and throbbing in the temples. The headaches are associated with nausea, vomiting to the point of dehydration, photophobia, phonophobia, and blurring of vision. They are preceded by confusion, irritability, lightheadedness, double vision, slurring of speech, and impaired coordination. These symptoms start 2–4 hours before the onset of headache and last for the duration of the headaches.

## MIMICS OF MIGRAINE WITH AURA

As described in Chapter 17 for migraine without aura, other conditions can also masquerade as migraine with aura. Because the aura of migraine is generally visual, these tend to be conditions of the visual system, most often the eye or occipital lobe. The following case studies are two examples of visual conditions mimicking migraine with aura, one related to the eye and the other to the occipital lobe.

A 25-year-old man has had headaches for 10 years. The headaches presently occur three to five times per month and usually start at the end of the morning. They start with tightening of the periorbital muscle on the right and reddening of the right eye. This is followed by blurring of vision in the right eye, which makes him feel nauseated and lightheaded. Within 1 hour, pain begins above the right eye, which in 10 minutes develops into a bifrontal headache. The headaches are moderate in intensity, throbbing, and associated with nausea and photophobia. Exertion and sudden movements make them worse and increase the throbbing. Lying down in a dark room and applying a cold compress to the forehead relieve the headaches somewhat. Reading, working at a computer terminal, and bright, especially fluorescent, or strobe light bring on headache. This is less likely to occur, however, if the patient consistently uses the glasses that he was prescribed for hyperopia.

---

A 51-year-old woman has had headaches since age 27 years. The headaches started after her second pregnancy. They have been severe since their onset but initially occurred infrequently (less than once per month). The headaches gradually increased in frequency and have been daily for the last 10 years. They are present on awakening in the morning 1–2 days per week but otherwise start at any time during the day. The headaches build to their maximum intensity in 20 minutes and last for 6 hours. They are located on the left, behind the eye and in the frontotemporal area. The headaches are throbbing and are associated with photophobia of both eyes. They are associated with nausea twice per week and with vomiting once per month. When the headaches begin during the day, they are preceded by a visual disturbance. The visual disturbance lasts for

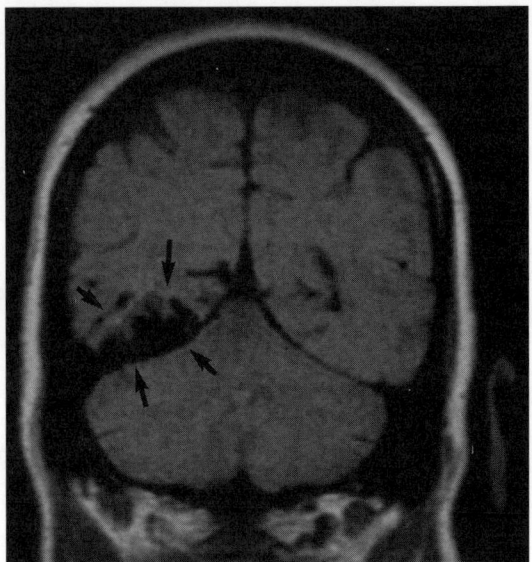

**Figure 18-5.** Magnetic resonance imaging shows an arteriovenous malformation of the left occipital lobe (arrows).

10–15 minutes and consists of black, vertical, squiggly lines that move downward across the right visual field. Magnetic resonance imaging revealed an arteriovenous malformation of the left occipital lobe (Fig. 18-5).

In the first of the preceding two case studies, the headaches were heralded by obvious symptoms of eyestrain—that is, contraction of the periorbital muscle, reddening of the eye, and blurring of vision in that eye. Blurring of vision, especially when it precedes the onset of headache, is often taken for an aura symptom. Aura symptoms of migraine are transient focal neurologic symptoms, however, and blurring of vision does not fall into that category. Blurring of vision is an ophthalmologic symptom and is generated in the eyeball. It is monocular, whereas the visual symptoms of the migraine aura are homonymous.

Blurring of vision is common with headaches, however, including migraine, although this is not generally appreciated. It most often occurs as an associated symptom of the headache, such as the nausea and vomiting of migraine. As with these gastrointestinal symptoms, it usually occurs only when the headaches are severe, and therefore it is more common in migraine than in tension-type headache. When blurring of vision occurs secondary to headache, it is probably due to weakening of the muscle(s) of accommodation, resulting from activation of the rudimentary sympathetic innervation of the muscle(s). When blurring of vision precedes the onset of headache, the muscle(s) of accommodation give way as a result of strain, whereas the muscle contraction resulting from the strain continues to build to the extent that headache develops.

## VISUAL SYMPTOMS AND EYESTRAIN

In a study, two colleagues and I looked at visual symptoms and eyestrain factors in 94 patients with chronic headache and compared them with 90 age- and gender-matched controls.[6] With regard to visual symptoms, we studied photophobia and blurring of vision. Photophobia was significantly more common in the headache patients than in the controls (45% versus 28%). Photophobia further increased to 71% in the headache patients when headache was actually present. Blurring of vision, on the other hand, was equally common in the two groups. However, blurring of vision was significantly more common in the headache patients when headache was present than in its absence (45% versus 7%). This means that almost half of the patients experienced blurring of vision with their headaches.

With regard to eyestrain factors, we looked at precipitation and aggravation of headache by bright light, reading, working at a computer, and watching television. The results are presented in Table 18-1. They show that aggravation of headache by eyestrain factors was very common and that 15% of the

**Table 18-1. Eyestrain factors in chronic headache (n = 94)**

| Factor | Precipitation of headache (% of patients) | Aggravation of headache (% of patients) |
|---|---|---|
| Bright light | 29 | 73 |
| Reading | 16 | 55 |
| Working at a computer | 14 | 31 |
| Watching television | 6 | 28 |

Source: Adapted from AJP Vincent, ELH Spierings, HB Messinger. A controlled study of visual symptoms and eye strain factors in chronic headache. Headache 1989;29:523–527.

chronic headache patients got headache from near-vision activities, such as reading and working at a computer.

In the second of the preceding two case studies, there was nothing unusual about the presentation of the headache or aura symptoms per se. What stood out as a red flag, however, was the fact that the headaches *always* occurred on the left and the aura symptoms *always* on the right. This is referred to as *crossed and fixed lateralization of the headache and aura*, which always requires further neurologic evaluation to rule out structural illness. It is reassuring with migraine to see symptoms that alternate sides as well as neurologic non-sense (e.g., a headache that is preceded by a visual disturbance on the same side [neurologic non-sense] as opposed to the other side [neurologic sense]), or both. Typically, with migraine, the headache occurs sometimes on the right and sometimes on the left, although often there is a preference for one side or the other. The aura symptoms alternate sides also, and it is further reassuring when this occurs independent of the headache.

## REFERENCES

1. Olesen J, Larsen B, Lauritzen M. Focal hyperemia followed by spreading oligemia and impaired activation of rCBF in classic migraine. Ann Neurol 1981;9:344–352.
2. Lauritzen M, Olsen TS, Lassen NA, Paulson OB. Changes in regional cerebral blood flow during the course of classic migraine attacks. Ann Neurol 1983;13:633–641.
3. Milner PM. Note on a possible correspondence between the scotomas of migraine and spreading depression of Leão. Electroencephalogr Clin Neurophysiol 1958;10:705.
4. Lauritzen M, Jørgensen MB, Diemer NH, et al. Persistent oligemia of rat cerebral cortex in the wake of spreading depression. Ann Neurol 1982;12:469–474.

5. Spierings ELH. Angiographic changes suggestive of vasospasm in migraine complicated by stroke. Headache 1990;30:727–728.
6. Vincent AJP, Spierings ELH, Messinger HB. A controlled study of visual symptoms and eye strain factors in chronic headache. Headache 1989;29: 523–527.

# Abortive Migraine Treatment

The treatment of migraine headache, like that of headaches in general, can be divided into abortive and preventive. Abortive treatment is *always* indicated when headaches are moderate or severe in intensity, as is generally the case with migraine. For the abortive treatment of migraine headache, analgesics and vasoconstrictors can be used. When these medications are taken by mouth, absorption must be considered. Dysfunction of the gastrointestinal tract during a migraine headache impairs the absorption of oral medications.[1] This dysfunction consists of atony and dilation of the stomach and closure of the pyloric sphincter (Fig. 19-1). The dysfunction results from activation of the sympathetic nervous system due to the pain of migraine headache.[2]

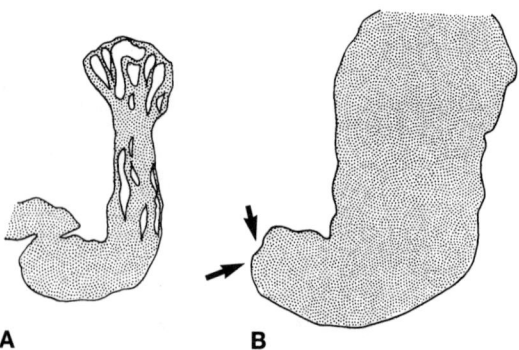

**A**        **B**

**Figure 19-1.** Upper gastrointestinal tract between (A) and during (B) migraine headache, shows atony and dilation of the stomach and closure of the pyloric sphincter (arrows) during the headache. (Adapted from J Kaufman, I Levine. Acute gastric dilatation of the stomach during attacks of migraine. Radiology 1936;27:301–302.)

## TREATMENT OF GASTROINTESTINAL DYSFUNCTION

The gastrointestinal dysfunction of migraine can be addressed with metoclopramide (Reglan), which is an antinausea medication with gastrokinetic properties. It stimulates the gastrointestinal tract and thereby corrects the impaired absorption of oral medications.[3] Metoclopramide is taken in a dose of

10 mg by mouth but must be taken early (i.e., at the onset of the headache) to be absorbed. It generally does not cause drowsiness or any other side effects and therefore can be taken early without problems. Medications for treatment of the headache are often more effective when taken 15 minutes after the metoclopramide.[4]

## TREATMENT OF PAIN WITH ORAL MEDICATIONS

A useful oral medication for treatment of migraine headache is Midrin, which is a combination of isometheptene, dichloralphenazone, and acetaminophen.[5] Isometheptene is an indirectly acting sympathomimetic with mild vasoconstrictor activity, and dichloralphenazone is a mild sedative. Midrin is generally well tolerated, with few if any side effects, of which the most common is stomach upset. It is taken in a dosage of two capsules at the onset of headache, followed by one capsule every half hour, with a maximum of six capsules per day. The medication is contraindicated with the concomitant use of a monoamine oxidase inhibitor.

A step up in potency from Midrin in the oral abortive treatment of migraine are the selective serotonin 1B/D receptor agonists. These medica-

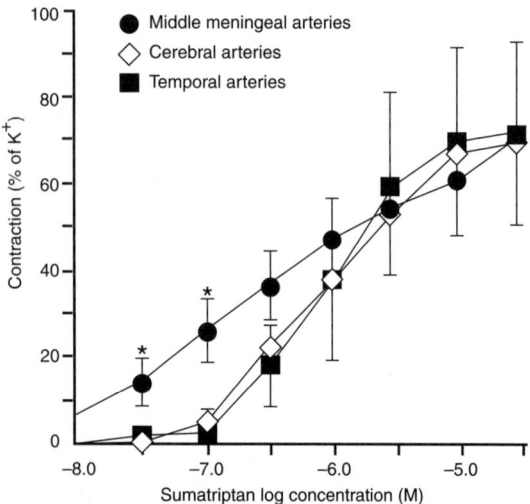

**Figure 19-2.** Effect of sumatriptan on the human meningeal, cerebral, and temporal arteries. (M = molar.) (Reprinted with permission from I Jansen, L Edvinsson, A Mortensen, J Olesen. Sumatriptan is a potent vasoconstrictor of human dural arteries via a 5-HT1–like receptor. Cephalalgia 1992;12:203.)

tions are collectively referred to as *tryptans*, but a more appropriate name might be *selective serotonin agonists*. They cause constriction of extracranial, meningeal, and cerebral arteries as is shown in Fig. 19-2 for sumatriptan.[6] They also inhibit the mechanism of neurogenic inflammation, which, together with vasodilation, is responsible for the pain of migraine headache.

## NEUROGENIC INFLAMMATION

*Neurogenic inflammation* refers to inflammation of peripheral tissue caused by the release of chemicals from the primary sensory nerve fibers involved in pain transmission. These chemicals, which include substance P, calcitonin gene–related peptide, and neurokinin A, are released from the nerve fibers when they are activated.

In migraine, vasodilation causes the activation of the nerve fibers. The nerve fibers coil around the arteries and are stretched when the blood vessels dilate. Stretching of the nerve fibers causes them to depolarize, which leads to the generation of action potentials and the release of the inflammatory chemicals mentioned in the previous paragraph. The action potentials are carried to the central nervous system, where they lead to the perception of pain. The chemicals cause an inflammatory reaction, which results in further dilation of the blood vessels. This reaction also causes a lowering of the pain threshold locally in the peripheral tissue, thereby augmenting the pain resulting from the vasodilation.

**Table 19-1. Selective serotonin agonists in development**

Almotriptan
Eletriptan
Frovatriptan
Rizatriptan

## SEROTONIN AGONISTS

The serotonin 1B/D agonists attack this vicious cycle of vasodilation and inflammation from two sides. By stimulating postsynaptic 1B receptors located on the vascular smooth muscle, they induce vasoconstriction. By stimulating presynaptic 1D receptors on the nerve fibers, the serotonin agonists inhibit the release of inflammatory chemicals.

Of the selective serotonin agonists, sumatriptan (Imitrex), zolmitriptan (Zomig), and naratriptan (Amerge) are available on the market while others are in development (Table 19-1).

### Sumatriptan

Sumatriptan is available in 25- and 50-mg tablets, and the dosage is 25–100 mg every 2 hours, with a maximum of 200 mg per day. The optimal dose, however, is 50 mg, which has been shown to provide the same headache relief as 100 mg and is tolerated as well as 25 mg in terms of adverse events

**Table 19-2. Efficacy and tolerability of sumatriptan, 25, 50, and 100 mg, versus placebo**

| Medication | Patients experiencing headache relief at 4 hrs (%) | Patients experiencing adverse events (%) |
|---|---|---|
| Placebo | 38 | 20 |
| Sumatriptan | | |
| 25 mg | 67 | 24 |
| 50 mg | 78 | 27 |
| 100 mg | 79 | 37 |

Source: Adapted from V Pfaffenrath. Efficacy and safety of sumatriptan tablets (25 mg, 50 mg, 100 mg) in the acute treatment of migraine: defining the optimal dose of oral sumatriptan [abstract]. Headache 1997;37:327.

(Table 19-2).[7] Headache relief is defined as a reduction in headache intensity from moderate or severe to mild or no headache at 4 hours of treatment.

The side effects of oral sumatriptan are generally mild and brief and mostly consist of numbness of the fingers and tightness of the throat. Sumatriptan is a potent vasoconstrictor and therefore is contraindicated in uncontrolled hypertension and coronary artery disease. It is contraindicated also with the concomitant use of a monoamine oxidase inhibitor.

## Zolmitriptan

Zolmitriptan is available in 2.5- and 5.0-mg tablets, and the dosage is 2.5–5.0 mg every 2 hours, with a

**Table 19-3. Efficacy of zolmitriptan, 2.5 and 5.0 mg, versus placebo**

| Medication | Patients experiencing headache relief at 2 hrs (%) | Patients experiencing headache relief at 4 hrs (%) |
|---|---|---|
| Placebo | 34 | 32 |
| Zolmitriptan | | |
| 2.5 mg | 65 | 75 |
| 5.0 mg | 67 | 77 |

Source: Adapted from AM Rapoport, NM Ramadan, JU Adelman, et al. Optimizing the dose of zolmitriptan (Zomig, 311C90) for the acute treatment of migraine. A multicenter, double-blind, placebo-controlled, dose range–finding study. Neurology 1997;49:1210–1218.

maximum of 10 mg per day. The efficacy of the medication in providing headache relief at 2 and 4 hours of treatment is shown in Table 19-3.[8]

As shown, the headache relief provided by zolmitriptan at 2 and 4 hours is virtually the same for the two doses. This is also true for 24-hour headache recurrence but not for the tolerability (i.e., the occurrence of adverse events), which is considerably higher with the 5.0-mg dose (Table 19-4). Hence, the optimal dose for zolmitriptan is 2.5 mg.

Compared to sumatriptan, 50 mg,[9] zolmitriptan, 2.5 mg, looks more effective in providing 2-hour headache relief (Table 19-5). Considering the difference in placebo response, however, the difference in efficacy becomes questionable.

**Table 19-4. Tolerability and headache recurrence of zolmitriptan, 2.5 and 5.0 mg**

| Medication | Patients experiencing adverse events (%) | Patients experiencing headache recurrence within 24 hrs (%) |
|---|---|---|
| Zolmitriptan | | |
| 2.5 mg | 44 | 37 |
| 5.0 mg | 58 | 32 |

Source: Adapted from AM Rapoport, NM Ramadan, JU Adelman, et al. Optimizing the dose of zolmitriptan (Zomig, 311C90) for the acute treatment of migraine. A multicenter, double-blind, placebo-controlled, dose range–finding study. Neurology 1997;49:1210–1218.

**Table 19-5. Efficacy of zolmitriptan, 2.5 mg, and sumatriptan, 50 mg, versus placebo**

| Medication | Patients experiencing headache relief at 2 hrs (%) | Patients experiencing placebo response (%) |
|---|---|---|
| Zolmitriptan, 2.5 mg[a] | 65 | 34 |
| Sumatriptan, 50 mg[b] | 54 | 17 |

[a]AM Rapoport, NM Ramadan, JU Adelman, et al. Optimizing the dose of zolmitriptan (Zomig, 311C90) for the acute treatment of migraine. A multicenter, double-blind, placebo-controlled, dose range–finding study. Neurology 1997;49:1210–1218.
[b]J Sargent, JR Kirchner, R Davis, B Kirkhart, et al. Oral sumatriptan is effective and well tolerated for the acute treatment of migraine: results of a multicenter study. Neurology 1995;45(suppl 7):10–14.

The most common side effects of zolmitriptan are dizziness, fatigue, drowsiness, paresthesias, and nausea.[8] The medication may have more central nervous system side effects than sumatriptan because it crosses the blood-brain barrier much more readily. Like sumatriptan, zolmitriptan is contraindicated in patients with uncontrolled hypertension or coronary artery disease, as well as with the concomitant use of a monoamine oxidase inhibitor.

## Naratriptan

Naratriptan is available in a 2.5-mg tablet, and the dosage is 2.5 mg. This dose can be repeated once in 24 hours, with a minimum interval of 4 hours. The efficacy of the medication in providing headache relief at 4 hours of treatment is 68%.[10] Naratriptan is somewhat less effective than sumatriptan, 50 mg[7] (Table 19-6).

Naratriptan seems to be relatively free of side effects.[10] It is also not contraindicated with the concomitant use of monoamine oxidase inhibitor. However, it is contraindicated in uncontrolled hypertension and coronary artery disease.

## Rizatriptan

Of the selective serotonin agonists in development, rizatriptan (Maxalt) is expected to come on the mar-

**Table 19-6. Efficacy of naratriptan, 2.5 mg, and sumatriptan, 50 mg, versus placebo**

| Medication | Patients experiencing headache relief at 4 hrs (%) | Patients experiencing placebo response (%) |
|---|---|---|
| Naratriptan, 2.5 mg[a] | 68 | 33 |
| Sumatriptan, 50 mg[b] | 78 | 38 |

[a]NT Mathew, M Asgharnejad, M Peykamian, et al. Naratriptan is effective and well tolerated in the acute treatment of migraine. Results of a double-blind, placebo-controlled, crossover study. Neurology 1997;49:1485–1490.
[b]V Pfaffenrath. Efficacy and safety of sumatriptan tablets (25 mg, 50 mg, 100 mg) in the acute treatment of migraine: defining the optimal dose of oral sumatriptan [abstract]. Headache 1997;37:327.

ket shortly. In a dose of 10 mg, this medication provides headache relief at 2 hours in 52% of patients.[11] This is approximately the same as the relief obtained with sumatriptan, 50 mg[9] (Table 19-7).

## Comparative Efficacy

On the basis of the results presented in the preceding sections, it seems that the selective serotonin agonists are equally effective in the dosages indicated, except for naratriptan, which is somewhat less effective. Apart from efficacy, it is also important, however, to consider tolerability and 24-hour headache recurrence—that is, the occurrence of moderate or severe headache after initial relief to mild or no headache

**Table 19-7. Efficacy of rizatriptan, 10 mg, and sumatriptan, 50 mg, versus placebo**

| Medication | Patients experiencing headache relief at 2 hrs (%) | Patients experiencing placebo response (%) |
|---|---|---|
| Rizatriptan, 10 mg[a] | 52 | 18 |
| Sumatriptan, 50 mg[b] | 54 | 17 |

[a]WH Visser, GM Terwindt, SA Reines, et al. Rizatriptan vs sumatriptan in the acute treatment of migraine. A placebo-controlled, dose-ranging study. Arch Neurol 1996;53:1132–1137.
[b]J Sargent, JR Kirchner, R Davis, B Kirkhart, et al. Oral sumatriptan is effective and well tolerated for the acute treatment of migraine: results of a multicenter study. Neurology 1995;45(suppl 7):10–14.

within 24 hours of treatment. Table 19-8 suggests that the medications are also comparable in these aspects, except for naratriptan, which has a somewhat lower headache recurrence rate.

## ALTERNATE ROUTES OF ADMINISTRATION

When oral medications fail to relieve migraine headache, impaired absorption is usually at fault. Rather than increasing the strength of the medication, it is generally more effective to alter the route of administration. Giving a medication other than by mouth is also more effective once the migraine headache has established itself, for example, when it is present on

**Table 19-8. Tolerability and headache recurrence of selective serotonin agonists**

| Medication | Patients experiencing adverse events (%) | Patients experiencing headache recurrence within 24 hrs (%) |
| --- | --- | --- |
| Naratriptan, 2.5 mg[a] | 31 | 27 |
| Rizatriptan, 10 mg[b] | 48 | 41 |
| Sumatriptan, 50 mg[c] | 37 | — |
| Zolmitriptan, 2.5 mg[d] | 44 | 36 |

[a]NT Mathew, M Asgharnejad, M Peykamian, et al. Naratriptan is effective and well tolerated in the acute treatment of migraine. Results of a double-blind, placebo-controlled, crossover study. Neurology 1997;49:1485–1490.

[b]WH Visser, GM Terwindt, SA Reines, et al. Rizatriptan vs sumatriptan in the acute treatment of migraine. A placebo-controlled, dose-ranging study. Arch Neurol 1996;53:1132–1137.

[c]J Sargent, JR Kirchner, R Davis, B Kirkhart, et al. Oral sumatriptan is effective and well tolerated for the acute treatment of migraine: results of a multicenter study. Neurology 1995;45(suppl 7):10–14.

[d]AM Rapoport, NM Ramadan, JU Adelman, et al. Optimizing the dose of zolmitriptan (Zomig, 311C90) for the acute treatment of migraine. A multicenter, double-blind, placebo-controlled, dose range–finding study. Neurology 1997;49:1210–1218.

awakening in the morning or when it wakes the patient up at night. An effective way of administering a medication under these circumstances is by nasal spray or rectal suppository. Injection offers another alternative.

## Nasal Spray

The nasal sprays that are available for the abortive treatment of migraine are sumatriptan and dihydroergotamine (Migranal). Dihydroergotamine, unlike sumatriptan, is a *non*selective serotonin 1B/D agonist, which means that it also interacts with many other receptors.[12]

### Sumatriptan

The sumatriptan nasal spray contains 20 mg of the medication per spray. This dose can be repeated once in 24 hours, with a minimum interval of 2 hours. The efficacy of the nasal spray in providing headache relief is 53% at 1 hour and 64% at 2 hours (Fig. 19-3).[13] The nasal spray provides the same headache relief in 2 hours as the 50-mg tablet does in 4 hours. This means that its onset of action is approximately twice as fast as the tablet. The most common side effect of the nasal spray is a bad or bitter taste in the mouth.

### Dihydroergotamine

The dihydroergotamine nasal spray is given in a dose of 2 mg, which is administered in four sprays, one in each nostril, repeated after 15 minutes. The efficacy of the nasal spray in providing headache relief is 63% at 2 hours and 70% at 4 hours (Fig. 19-4).[14] Its most common side effect is nasal congestion, followed by a bad taste in the mouth and nausea.

Like sumatriptan, dihydroergotamine is a potent arterial vasoconstrictor and is therefore contraindi-

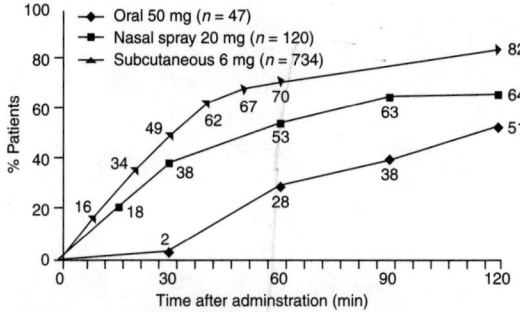

**Figure 19-3.** Efficacy of sumatriptan given orally, nasally, and subcutaneously in the abortive treatment of migraine, defined as a reduction in headache intensity from moderate or severe to mild or no headache. (Reprinted with permission from C Dahlof. Would any acute treatment for migraine demonstrate recurrence? Cephalalgia 1997;17[suppl 17]:19.)

cated in patients with uncontrolled hypertension or coronary artery disease.

The 24-hour recurrence of headache with the dihydroergotamine nasal spray is 15%.[14] This is considerably lower than the recurrence rate seen with sumatriptan, whether administered orally, nasally, or by subcutaneous injection. The 24-hour headache recurrence rate of sumatriptan is approximately 35%, which means that one-third of patients experience recurrence of headache within 24 hours after admin-

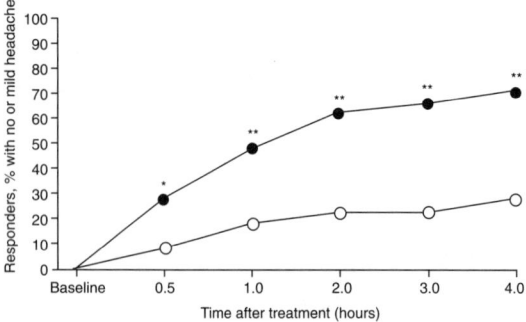

**Figure 19-4.** Efficacy of dihydroergotamine, 2 mg nasally (closed circles), versus placebo (open circles) in the abortive treatment of migraine. (Reprinted with permission from RM Gallagher for the Dihydroergotamine Working Group. Acute treatment of migraine with dihydroergotamine nasal spray. Arch Neurol 1996;53:1288.)

istration of the medication. The medication can, of course, be repeated at this time, but if this is a pattern, a medication with a lower recurrence rate can be used, such as the dihydroergotamine nasal spray.

## Rectal Suppository

The rectal suppositories that can be used for the abortive treatment of migraine are indomethacin (Indocin) and ergotamine with caffeine (Cafergot).

## Indomethacin

Indomethacin is a potent anti-inflammatory analgesic with mild constrictor effect on the extracranial and cerebral arteries.[15] It is available as a suppository in a dose of 50 mg, of which one can be taken every half hour, with a maximum of four per day.[16] The most common side effect of the medication is orthostatic lightheadedness, caused by its general vasodilator effect. Indomethacin is contraindicated in patients with peptic ulcer disease or bleeding disorder.

## Ergotamine

Ergotamine is, as is dihydroergotamine, a nonselective serotonin agonist. The ergotamine with caffeine suppository contains 2 mg ergotamine combined with 100 mg caffeine to improve absorption. In a dose of 1 mg (one-half of a suppository), ergotamine has been shown to relieve a migraine headache within 3 hours in 73% of patients.[17] Nausea and vomiting are its most common side effects, and therefore it is important to administer the medication with care. I usually advise patients to take only one-fourth or one-third of a suppository at a time and to repeat that, if necessary, every 30–60 minutes, with a maximum of two suppositories per day. When taken in this way, the ergotamine with caffeine suppository often provides effective relief of migraine headaches without causing significant gastrointestinal side effects. It can also be combined with an antinausea medication, either orally or rectally, to treat the gastrointestinal side effects. As are the selective serotonin agonists and dihydroergotamine, ergotamine is a potent vasoconstrictor and is contraindicated in uncontrolled hypertension and coronary artery disease.

Ergotamine is a long-acting medication, and its vasoconstrictor effect has been shown to last for at least 3 days.[18] This means that it should not be used more often than once per week. If used more frequently than that, the wearing off of the medication's effect is followed by rebound vasodilation and headache that is indistinguishable from migraine. A cycle is thus created in which the occurrence of headache and intake of ergotamine gradually increase over time, ultimately leading to an intractable condition in which headaches occur frequently, requiring daily or almost daily use of ergotamine. The only way this condition can be treated is by total discontinuation of the medication, for which hospitalization may be required. Once the withdrawal has been accomplished, a dramatic reduction in the frequency of migraine headaches usually follows.[19]

## Injection

Another route of administering a medication for the abortive treatment of migraine is by injection. The injection of dihydroergotamine (D.H.E. 45) and sumatriptan (Imitrex) in the context of the treatment of acute, severe headache is discussed in Chapter 6. Sumatriptan is also available with an autoinjector for easy subcutaneous administration by patients themselves at home. For this purpose, it is available in pre-filled syringes that contain 6 mg of the medication. Self-injected sumatriptan has been shown to be 77% effective in decreasing the intensity of moderate or severe headache to mild or no headache within 1 hour of treatment.[20] The most common side effects of sumatriptan taken by injection are lightheadedness and a hot, tight, or tingling sensation, generally in the upper chest, anterior neck, and face.

The sumatriptan injection can be repeated, if necessary, after 1 hour, but it has been shown that this does *not* increase its efficacy. Also, administration of sumatriptan by injection during the migraine aura has been shown *not* to affect the ensuing headache.[21] However, administration of the medication during the aura is safe and does not affect the intensity or duration of the aura symptoms.

Medications that are effective in the abortive treatment of migraine are summarized in Table 19-9.

**Table 19-9. Summary of the abortive treatment of migraine**

| Route of administration | Medication | Dosage | Side effects | Contraindications |
|---|---|---|---|---|
| Oral | Isomethep-tene | Two capsules at the onset, followed by one capsule every half hr; maximum six capsules/day | Drowsiness; rest-lessness; stomach upset | Use of a mono-amine oxidase inhibitor |
| | Sumatriptan | 25–100 mg as needed every 2 hrs; maximum 200 mg/day | Numbness in the fingers; tightness of the throat | Uncontrolled hypertension; coronary artery disease; use of a monoamine oxidase inhibitor |
| | Zolmitriptan | 2.5–5.0 mg as needed every 2 hrs; maximum 10 mg/day | Dizziness; fatigue; drowsiness; pares-thesias; nausea | Uncontrolled hypertension; coronary artery disease; use of a monoamine oxidase inhibitor |
| | Naratriptan | 2.5 mg; can be repeated after 4 hrs; maximum 5 mg/day | | Uncontrolled hypertension; coronary artery disease |

| | | | | |
|---|---|---|---|---|
| Nasal | Sumatriptan | 20 mg; can be repeated after 2 hrs; maximum two sprays/day | Bad or bitter taste in the mouth | Uncontrolled hypertension; coronary artery disease |
| | Dihydroergotamine | 2 mg in four sprays over 15 mins | Nasal congestion; bad taste in the mouth; nausea | Uncontrolled hypertension; coronary artery disease |
| Rectal | Indomethacin | 50 mg every half hr; maximum 200 mg/day | Orthostatic lightheadedness | Peptic ulcer disease; bleeding disorder |
| | Ergotamine | One-fourth or one-third suppository as needed every half hr to 1 hr; maximum two suppositories/day | Nausea; vomiting; leg cramp | Uncontrolled hypertension; coronary artery disease |
| Parenteral | Sumatriptan | 6 mg; can be repeated after 1 hr; maximum two injections/day | Tingling; chest tightness; lightheadedness | Uncontrolled hypertension; coronary artery disease |
| | Dihydroergotamine | 1 mg; can be repeated after 1 hr; maximum two injections/day | Nausea; vomiting | Uncontrolled hypertension; coronary artery disease |

# REFERENCES

1. Volans GN. Absorption of effervescent aspirin during migraine. BMJ 1974;4:265–269.
2. Anthony M. Biochemical indices of sympathetic activity in migraine. Cephalalgia 1981;1:83–89.
3. Volans GN. The effect of metoclopramide on the absorption of effervescent aspirin in migraine. Br J Clin Pharmacol 1975;2:57–63.
4. Tfelt-Hansen P, Olesen J. Effervescent metoclopramide and aspirin (Migravess) versus effervescent aspirin or placebo for migraine attacks: a double-blind study. Cephalalgia 1984;4:107–111.
5. Diamond S. Treatment of migraine with isometheptene, acetaminophen, and dichloralphenazone combination: a double-blind, crossover trial. Headache 1976;15:282–287.
6. Jansen I, Edvinsson L, Mortensen A, Olesen J. Sumatriptan is a potent vasoconstrictor of human dural arteries via a 5-HT$_1$-like receptor. Cephalalgia 1992;12:202–205.
7. Pfaffenrath V. Efficacy and safety of sumatriptan tablets (25 mg, 50 mg, 100 mg) in the acute treatment of migraine: defining the optimal dose of oral sumatriptan [abstract]. Headache 1997;37:327.
8. Rapoport AM, Ramadan NM, Adelman JU, et al. Optimizing the dose of zolmitriptan (Zomig, 311C90) for the acute treatment of migraine. A multicenter, double-blind, placebo-controlled, dose range–finding study. Neurology 1997;49:1210–1218.
9. Sargent J, Kirchner JR, Davis R, Kirkhart B. Oral sumatriptan is effective and well tolerated for the

acute treatment of migraine: results of a multicenter study. Neurology 1995;45(suppl 7):10–14.

10. Mathew NT, Asgharnejad M, Peykamian M, et al. Naratriptan is effective and well tolerated in the acute treatment of migraine. Results of a double-blind, placebo-controlled, crossover study. Neurology 1997;49:1485–1490.

11. Visser WH, Terwindt GM, Reines SA, et al. Rizatriptan vs sumatriptan in the acute treatment of migraine. A placebo-controlled, dose-ranging study. Arch Neurol 1996;53:1132–1137.

12. McCarthy BG, Peroutka SJ. Comparative neuropharmacology of dihydroergotamine and sumatriptan (GR 43175). Headache 1989;29:420–422.

13. Dahlof C. Would any acute treatment for migraine demonstrate recurrence? Cephalalgia 1997;17 (suppl 17):17–20.

14. Gallagher RM for the Dihydroergotamine Working Group. Acute treatment of migraine with dihydroergotamine nasal spray. Arch Neurol 1996;53: 1285–1291.

15. Sicuteri F, Michelacci S, Anselmi B. Termination of migraine headache by a new anti-inflammatory vasoconstrictor agent. Clin Pharmacol Ther 1965;6: 336–344.

16. Nelemans F. Een technisch gelukt onderzoek met indomethacine bij patienten lijdende aan migraine. Een dubbelblind onderzoek versus placebo. Huisarts Wetenschap 1971;14:337–340.

17. Graham JR. Rectal use of ergotamine tartrate and caffeine alkaloid for the relief of migraine. N Engl J Med 1954;250:936–938.

18. Tfelt-Hansen P, Paalzow L. Intramuscular ergota-

mine: plasma levels and dynamic activity. Clin Pharmacol Ther 1985;37:29–35.

19. Tfelt-Hansen P, Aebelholt Krabbe A. Ergotamine abuse. Do patients benefit from withdrawal? Cephalalgia 1981;1:29–32.

20. Sumatriptan Auto-Injector Study Group. Self-treatment of acute migraine with subcutaneous sumatriptan using an auto-injector device. Eur Neurol 1991;31:323–331.

21. Bates D, Ashford E, Dawson R, et al. Subcutaneous sumatriptan during the migraine aura. Neurology 1994;44:1587–1592.

# Preventive Migraine Treatment

When migraine headaches occur frequently (i.e., more than twice per month), preventive treatment may be indicated. Preventive treatment may also be indicated when the headaches are intense or prolonged or when abortive treatment is ineffective.

The medications that have been shown to be effective in the preventive treatment of migraine are methysergide (Sansert),[1–3] the beta-blockers that lack partial agonist or intrinsic sympathomimetic activity,[4] amitriptyline (Elavil),[5, 6] verapamil (Isoptin),[7, 8] and valproate (Depakote)[9–11] (Table 20-1).

**Table 20-1. Medications effective in the preventive treatment of migraine**

Methysergide
Beta-blockers
    Atenolol
    Nadolol
    Metoprolol
    Propranolol
    Timolol
Amitriptyline
Verapamil
Valproate

## METHYSERGIDE

Methysergide is a mild vasoconstrictor and is available in 2-mg tablets. Treatment is usually initiated with a dosage of one tablet twice daily, after which it is increased to one tablet four times per day. The medication is given in divided doses because of its relatively short duration of action. It is taken with meals and at bedtime with food because it can cause nausea and indigestion. With long-term use, methysergide can give rise to retroperitoneal, pleuropulmonary, or endocardial fibrosis.[12, 13] Therefore, it should not be taken for longer than 4–6 months, after which it is discontinued for 2–4 weeks. The medication is contraindicated in hypertension, vascular disease, valvular heart disease, chronic pulmonary disease, collagen disease, and fibrotic conditions.

---

## BETA-BLOCKERS

---

The beta-blockers that lack partial agonist activity are atenolol (Tenormin), metoprolol (Lopressor), nadolol (Corgard), propranolol (Inderal), and timolol (Blocadren). These particular beta-blockers increase peripheral vascular resistance by increasing blood vessel tone, thereby mitigating the migrainous vasodilation.

### Propranolol

Propranolol is most commonly used for migraine prevention, generally in doses ranging from 80 to 160 mg per day. When the long-acting capsule is used, the medication can be given once daily. Side effects of propranolol are fatigue, depression, insomnia, and impotence. The medication is contraindicated in sinus bradycardia, atrioventricular block, congestive heart failure, obstructive pulmonary disease, and diabetes mellitus.

### Atenolol and Metoprolol

I prefer to prescribe atenolol or metoprolol over propranolol because they are often better tolerated and are equally effective. Both medications are long-acting and therefore can be given once daily. I usually initiate treatment with 25 mg atenolol or 50 mg metoprolol per day, after which I gradually increase the dosage. While increasing the dosage, I monitor the effect of the medication in decreasing the pulse rate. The decrease in pulse rate reflects the extent of beta-blockade achieved and I bring the pulse rate down, if necessary, to 50 or 60 beats per minute.

## AMITRIPTYLINE

Amitriptyline is a serotonin reuptake inhibitor that increases the pain threshold. It is best prescribed once daily at bedtime because it causes sedation. I usually initiate treatment with 25 mg and gradually increase the dose until some dryness of the mouth occurs. This medication is particularly helpful for patients who also have problems falling asleep or sleeping through the night. Apart from sedation and dry mouth, amitriptyline can cause constipation and weight gain. The medication is contraindicated in glaucoma, prostate hypertrophy, epilepsy, and cardiac arrhythmias.

## VERAPAMIL

Verapamil is a calcium-entry blocker that also increases the pain threshold.[14] I usually prescribe the 240-mg, sustained-release tablet, which can be given twice daily. I initiate treatment with a dose of 240 mg per day, after which I increase it to 480 mg per day. Verapamil is generally well tolerated, with constipation being its most common side effect. It is contraindicated in atrioventricular block and sick sinus syndrome because it slows down atrioventricular conduction.

## VALPROATE

Valproate is a gamma-aminobutyric acid–receptor agonist and antiepileptic medication. It is usually prescribed in dosages ranging from 500 to 1,500 mg per day in two to four administrations. It tends to cause nausea and indigestion and is therefore best taken with meals and at bedtime with food. The serum level can be determined and should preferably be maintained between 50 and 100 µg per ml. Liver function should also be determined regularly because of hepatotoxicity. Valproate is contraindicated in liver disease or when liver function is abnormal.

**Table 20-2. Rounded estimates of the efficacy of preventive antimigraine medications**

| Medication | Efficacy (%) |
|---|---|
| Methysergide, 6 mg/day | 55 |
| Beta-blockers | |
|     Atenolol, 100 mg/day | 50 |
|     Metoprolol, 100–200 mg/day | 50 |
|     Nadolol, 80–240 mg/day | 70 |
|     Propranolol, 80–160 mg/day | 55 |
|     Timolol, 10 mg twice daily | 50 |
| Amitriptyline, 10–150 mg/day | 60 |
| Verapamil, 80 mg three or four times/day | 50 |
| Valproate, 800–1,500 mg/day | 55 |

Source: Adapted from ELH Spierings. Management of Migraine. Boston: Butterworth–Heinemann, 1996;95.

## EFFICACY

Table 20-2 provides rounded estimates of the efficacy of preventive antimigraine medications.[15] The medications are roughly equally effective (50–60%, except for nadolol) in reducing headache frequency. Verapamil is probably the best tolerated, but in my experience it is not very effective, at least in migraine. Its effect on cluster headache is far better, and I consider it the preventive medication of choice for that condition (see Chapter 23). The beta-blockers are the next best tolerated and are generally more effective in migraine prevention than verapamil. Valproate tends to be poorly tolerated and, at least in my experience, no more effective than verapamil.

In preventive treatment of migraine, the physician should *always* try a single medication first. Medications can also be combined, however, and a good combination is that of a beta-blocker with amitriptyline. Special care should be taken when a beta-blocker is combined with methysergide because of peripheral vasoconstriction. Similarly, a beta-blocker combined with verapamil can cause bradycardia.

Of the selective serotonin reuptake inhibitors, fluoxetine (Prozac) and fluvoxamine (Luvox) have been studied in the preventive treatment of migraine. Fluoxetine was found to be effective in one study[16] but not in another, much larger study.[17] In a comparative trial, fluvoxamine reduced headache frequency from placebo baseline by 56%.[18]

The medications that are effective in the preventive treatment of migraine are summarized in Table 20-3.

**Table 20-3. Summary of the preventive treatment of migraine**

| Medication | Dosage | Side effects | Contraindications |
|---|---|---|---|
| Methysergide | 2 mg two to four times/day | Nausea; indigestion; fibrosis | Hypertension; vascular disease; valvular heart disease; chronic pulmonary disease; collagen disease; fibrotic conditions |
| Propranolol | 80–160 mg LA once daily | Fatigue; depression; insomnia; impotence | Sinus bradycardia; atrioventricular block; congestive heart failure; obstructive pulmonary disease; diabetes mellitus |
| Amitriptyline | 25–75 mg once daily at bedtime | Dry mouth; constipation; weight gain | Glaucoma; prostate hypertrophy; epilepsy; cardiac arrhythmias |
| Verapamil | 120–240 mg SR twice daily | Constipation | Atrioventricular block; sick sinus syndrome |
| Valproate | 500–1,500 mg/day | Nausea; indigestion; sedation | Abnormal liver function; liver disease |

LA = long acting; SR = sustained release.

# REFERENCES

1. Shekelle RB, Ostfeld AM. Methysergide in the migraine syndrome. Clin Pharmacol Ther 1964;5:201–204.
2. Southwell N, Williams JD, Mackenzie I. Methysergide in the prophylaxis of migraine. Lancet 1964;1:523–524.
3. Pedersen E, Møller CE. Methysergide in migraine prophylaxis. Clin Pharmacol Ther 1966;7:520–526.
4. Weerasuriya K, Patel L, Turner P. Beta-adrenoceptor blockade and migraine. Cephalalgia 1982;2:33–45.
5. Gomersall JD, Stuart A. Amitriptyline in migraine prophylaxis. Changes in pattern of attacks during a controlled clinical trial. J Neurol Neurosurg Psychiatry 1973;36:684–690.
6. Couch JR, Hassanein RS. Amitriptyline in migraine prophylaxis. Arch Neurol 1979;36:695–699.
7. Solomon GD, Steel JG, Spaccavento LJ. Verapamil prophylaxis of migraine. A double-blind, placebo-controlled study. JAMA 1983;250:2500–2502.
8. Markley HG, Cheroms JCD, Piepho RW. Verapamil in prophylactic therapy of migraine. Neurology 1984;34:973–976.
9. Hering R, Kuritzky A. Sodium valproate in the prophylactic treatment of migraine: a double-blind study versus placebo. Cephalalgia 1992;12:81–84.
10. Jensen R, Brinck T, Olesen J. Sodium valproate has a prophylactic effect in migraine without aura: a triple-blind, placebo-controlled cross-over study. Neurology 1994;44:647–651.

11. Mathew NT, Saper JR, Silberstein SD, et al. Migraine prophylaxis with divalproex. Arch Neurol 1995;52:281–286.
12. Graham JR. Methysergide for prevention of migraine. Experience in five hundred patients over three years. N Engl J Med 1964;270:67–72.
13. Graham JR. Cardiac and pulmonary fibrosis during methysergide therapy for headache. Am J Med Sci 1967;254:23–34.
14. Miranda HF, Bustamanta D, Kramer V, et al. Antinociceptive effects of $Ca^{2+}$ channel blockers. Eur J Pharmacol 1992;217:137–141.
15. Spierings ELH. Management of Migraine. Boston: Butterworth–Heinemann, 1996.
16. Adly C, Straumanis J, Chesson A. Fluoxetine prophylaxis of migraine. Headache 1992;32:101–104.
17. Saper JR, Silberstein SD, Lake AE, Winters ME. Double-blind trial of fluoxetine: chronic daily headache and migraine. Headache 1994;43:497–502.
18. Bank J. A comparative study of amitriptyline and fluvoxamine in migraine prophylaxis. Headache 1994;34:476–478.

# CHAPTER TWENTY-ONE

# Chronic Daily Headache

A 41-year-old woman has had headaches since age 8 years. Until 10 years ago, the headaches occurred once every 2–3 months and lasted for 1–2 days. They were severe in intensity and associated with nausea and vomiting. Ten years ago, she went back to work as a teacher when her husband started his own business. The headaches increased in frequency due to the resulting stress and became daily over 2 years. The headaches are present on awakening in the morning and are worst at that time. They wake her out of sleep at night 3 days per week on average. The headaches are moderate in intensity two or three times per month for 4–5 days and are severe once per month (with menstrual periods) for

5–6 days. The moderately intense headaches are generally located on the right but sometimes on the left, in the temple, as a throbbing pain. The severe headaches are located across the forehead from temple to temple. The headaches are associated with photophobia and, when severe, also with nausea, vomiting, and phonophobia. During the severe headaches, her hands and feet are very cold. Light and any kind of physical activity make the headaches worse. Lying down, applying ice to the forehead, and warming the hands and feet make them somewhat better. She generally feels very tired even though she sleeps well at night. Her neck and shoulder muscles are tight as well as sore to the extent of burning, more so on the left than on the right.

## PRESENTATION

*Chronic daily headache* refers to the daily or almost daily occurrence of headache for a lengthy period of time. In a recent study, several colleagues and I defined the condition as headaches occurring at least 5 days per week for at least 1 year.[1,2] The study examined the presentation and development of chronic daily headache in 258 patients (50 men and 208 women) whose headaches I had evaluated. The average age of the patients at the time of consultation was slightly older than 40 years. More than 75% of the patients had experienced the onset of headaches before age 30 years. Onset occurred more commonly in the second decade of life in women than in men (36% versus 24%), which is compatible with the importance of the onset of menstruation in headache in women.

## DIURNAL PATTERN

In almost 80% of the patients, the headaches were present on awakening in the morning or began in the course of the morning. In the remaining patients, the headaches began in the afternoon or evening or had a variable onset. In more than half of the patients, the headaches were at their worst in the afternoon or evening, and in one-fourth, they were worst on awakening or in the morning.

These results agree with my clinical observation that daily headaches come in two diurnal patterns. The most common pattern is that in which the headaches gradually increase in intensity as the day progresses, becoming worst in the afternoon. In the less common pattern, which I refer to as the *reversed diurnal pattern*, the headaches are worst on awakening in the morning and gradually improve as the day progresses. This is the pattern that the patient in the preceding case study describes.

The reversed diurnal pattern is particularly associated with the overuse of analgesics and vasoconstrictors. The severe headaches on awakening in the morning are caused by the withdrawal of medication overnight, and the gradual improvement during the day by the resumption of medication intake. This scenario is associated with the most frequent nighttime awakenings with headache. In the study, one-third of the patients were wakened at night by headache at least once per week. Of the patients wakened at least once per week by headache, 48% experienced their worst headaches on awakening or in the morning, as opposed to 22% of patients who were wakened by headache less than once per week.

## SEVERE HEADACHES

More than 90% of the patients in the study experienced severe headaches in addition to the daily headaches. One-fourth of the patients experienced severe headaches more than 15 days per month. This means that the majority of the patients with this condition, at least of those who seek specialty care for their headaches, do not have chronic tension-type headache. They have what I referred to in Chapter 14 as *tension-type vascular headache.* In patients who developed this condition out of migraine, as in the preceding case study, it could justifiably be called *chronic migraine.* However, not all patients develop the condition out of migraine, as the next case study illustrates.

---

A 54-year-old woman has had headaches since her teens. Initially, the headaches occurred two or three times per week and lasted for 5–6 hours. The headaches were located in one temple or the other, without preference, as a dull ache. They were not associated with nausea or vomiting and were relieved by nonprescription analgesics. The headaches gradually increased in frequency and have been daily for decades. They are present on awakening in the morning and gradually build in intensity as the day progresses, becoming worst in the early afternoon. The headaches do not wake her out of sleep at night. They are located on top of the head as a pressure. The headaches have been severe every day for the last 4–5 years. The severe headaches have also gradually increased in frequency and are associated with photophobia, phonophobia, and nausea. Becoming upset or nervous and experiencing tension make the headaches worse. Being very quiet and lying down make them somewhat

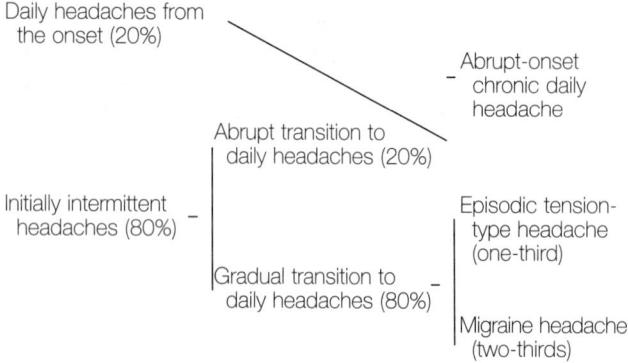

**Figure 21-1.** Development of chronic daily headache with the percentage of patients in each group.

better. Before menopause, the headaches were also worse with menstrual periods.

## SECONDARY CHRONIC DAILY HEADACHE

In 80% of the patients in the study described under Presentation, the daily headaches gradually developed out of initially intermittent headaches (Fig. 21-1). This could be called *secondary chronic daily headache*, in the same way we speak of primary and secondary chronic cluster headache (see Chapter 22).

In the two patients described in the preceding case studies, the daily headaches also developed gradually out of initially intermittent headaches. In the first patient, the intermittent headaches were severe and were associated with nausea and vomiting, compatible with migraine. In the second patient, the initial headaches were mild and were not associated with gastrointestinal symptoms, compatible with tension-type headache.

Of the patients in the study with secondary chronic daily headache *with gradual transition*, one-third initially experienced mild headaches and two-thirds had severe headaches. The mild headaches were associated with nausea in one-fourth of the patients but never with vomiting, whereas the severe headaches were associated with nausea or vomiting in the majority of the patients. The features of the daily headaches that the patients ultimately developed were the same, however, whether the initial headaches were mild or severe. The transition from intermittent to daily headaches was truly gradual, requiring a decade on average.

## PRIMARY CHRONIC DAILY HEADACHE

Twenty percent of the patients in the study had daily headaches from the onset (i.e., *primary chronic daily headache*), as the following case study illustrates.

---

A 14-year-old girl has had headaches since a flu at age 8 years. The flu was associated with severe headache, abdominal pain, and fatigue. The headaches have been daily since their onset. Until 6 months ago, the headaches started in the afternoon. Since that time, the headaches have been present on awakening in the morning and have also been more intense. They gradually build in intensity as the day progresses, becoming worst in the afternoon. The headaches are generally somewhat better again in the evening, and they do not wake her up at night. The headaches are located across the forehead and in the temples as a throbbing pain. They are associated with nausea and, when severe, also with photophobia and phonophobia. The headaches are severe 3–4 days per week. Light, noise, physical activity, and sometimes bending over make them worse. The headaches are also worse perimenstrually. Lying down makes them somewhat better. She has felt tired for the last 3 years. Her neck, shoulder, and jaw muscles are sore but not tight.

---

In our study, two-thirds of the patients with primary chronic daily headache experienced the onset of headaches in the second through fourth decade of life. In one-third, the onset of headaches occurred without apparent reason. In one-fourth, the onset of headaches was the result of a head, neck, or back injury and, in another one-fourth, headache onset resulted from illness or surgery.

With regard to the circumstances of headache onset and the features of the daily headaches, the group of patients with primary chronic daily headache was very similar to that of the patients with secondary chronic daily headache with abrupt transition. The two groups were therefore combined under the term *abrupt-onset chronic daily headache* (see Fig. 21-1). Twenty percent of the patients in this combined group had a prior history of severe headaches, which is also the prevalence of severe headaches in the United States population.[3] Therefore, it is clearly not necessary to have severe, albeit intermittent, headaches to develop daily headaches after an injury, illness, or surgery—a conclusion that may be important legally.

The occurrence of headache in the parents of patients was significantly more common in the gradual-onset group (69%) than in the abrupt-onset group (45%). In general, conditions that develop gradually have a greater genetic component than those that develop abruptly. Judging from the parental occurrence of headache, the pattern may also hold for chronic daily headache.

## REFERENCES

1. Spierings ELH, Schroevers M, Honkoop PC, Sorbi M. Presentation of chronic daily headache: a clinical study. Headache 1998;38:(in press).
2. Spierings ELH, Schroevers M, Honkoop PC, Sorbi M. Development of chronic daily headache: a clinical study. Headache 1998;38:(in press).
3. Celentano DD, Stewart WF, Lipton RB, Reed ML. Medication use and disability among migraineurs: a national probability sample survey. Headache 1992;32:223–228.

# Cluster Headache

A 25-year-old man has had headaches since age 15 years. The headaches occur in episodes lasting for 2 months. The episodes occur every 8–16 months. During the episodes, the headaches occur two or three times per day on average. One or two of the headaches wake him out of sleep at night, usually between 2 and 4 AM. The headaches build to their maximum intensity in 5–10 minutes and last for 45–60 minutes. They are excruciatingly severe and make him get out of bed and pace the floor. The headaches are located on the left and come up out of the back of the neck. They extend from there over the ear into the temple and the eye. The headaches are most intense in the eye, where they feel as if a hot poker is stuck through it. The eye tears, the ipsilateral nostril runs, and the temporal artery stands out prominently in the affected temple. Furthermore, the headaches are associated with mild nausea, phonophobia, and photophobia, with blurring of vision in the left eye. Pacing the floor and applying pressure to the left eye and temple make them somewhat better. Alcohol, daytime napping, smoke, hot dogs, and nuts bring on headache.

## PREVALENCE

Cluster headache is a chronic headache condition related to migraine but is much less common than migraine. Its prevalence in the general population is estimated at 70 per 100,000, with a male-to-female ratio of 14 to 1.[1]

## PRESENTATION

The clinical presentation of cluster headache is fairly constant (Table 22-1). Therefore, the condition is relatively easy to diagnose.

The headaches of cluster headache last from 30 minutes to 2 hours and occur once or twice per day. They tend to occur during the early night, waking

**Table 22-1. Clinical characteristics of cluster headache**

| Characteristic | Finding |
|---|---|
| Age of onset | 20–40 years old |
| Sex distribution | 90% male |
| Episodic | 85% of patients |
| Chronic | |
|     Primary | 10% of patients |
|     Secondary | 5% of patients |
| Attack duration | 30 mins to 2 hrs |
| Attack frequency | One to two/day |
| Duration of episodes | 2 wks to 2 mos |
| Duration of remissions | 6 mos to 1 yr |
| Laterality | |
|     Right | 50% of patients |
|     Left | 40% of patients |
|     Either | 10% of patients |
| Local autonomic symptoms | |
|     Ocular (tearing, reddening) | 80% of patients |
|     Nasal (running, stuffiness) | 70% of patients |
| Triggers | Alcohol; daytime napping |
| Family history | |
|     Cluster headache | 5% of patients |
|     Migraine | 40% of patients |

Source: Adapted from L Kudrow. Cluster Headache. New York: Oxford University Press, 1980.

the patient out of sleep 1–2 hours after retiring. In 85% of patients, the headaches occur in episodes (as in the preceding case study) lasting from 2 weeks to 2 months, separated by remissions of 6 months to 1 year. In the remaining 15% of patients, the headaches occur for longer than 1 year without remission. In these cases, the condition is referred to as *chronic*, as opposed to *episodic*, cluster headache. Of the patients with chronic cluster headache, 5% first experience the headaches in episodes and are considered to have secondary chronic cluster headache. The remaining 10% have primary chronic cluster headache—that is, they never experience headaches in episodes. The following case study is an example of a patient with primary chronic cluster headache.

---

A 20-year-old man has had headaches for 2 years. Initially, the headaches occurred once per month, but they gradually increased in frequency. For the last 9–10 months, the headaches have occurred daily, two to five times per day, with an average of three headaches per day. The headaches usually start during the day between 11 AM and 8 PM. Sometimes, however, they occur at night, waking him out of sleep between midnight and 2 AM. The headaches build to their maximum intensity in 20–25 minutes and last for 2 hours. They disappear more quickly than they start (i.e., in 5–10 minutes). The headaches are generally moderate in intensity but are severe every 2–3 days. They are very severe once every 1–2 weeks. With the severe headaches, he is incapacitated and feels restless. When they are very severe, he becomes agitated and paces the floor or runs around. The headaches are located behind the left eye and are very sharp. They are associated with phonophobia and with photophobia of the left eye. When severe or very severe, the headaches are also associated with nausea.

## CLUSTER SYMPTOMS

For the majority of patients, the onset of cluster headache occurs in the second to fourth decade of life. The pain of cluster headache is *always* unilateral. In 90% of patients, cluster headache always affects the same side of the head, with a slight preference for the right. The pain is usually located in or behind the eye, in the forehead, or in the temple. In these areas, autonomic symptoms often occur, such as reddening and tearing of the eye, edematous swelling and drooping of the upper eyelid, narrowing of the pupil, increased sweating over the forehead, and stuffiness and running of the nose. In general, these symptoms occur only on the side of the headaches and only during the presence of pain. The symptoms are *not* pathognomonic of cluster headache, however, and their presence is not required for the diagnosis. Systemic symptoms (e.g., nausea or vomiting) that are common in migraine are rare in cluster headache. Another prominent distinction between cluster headache and migraine is the behavior of the patient. Whereas patients with migraine usually lie down during the headache, patients with cluster headache typically pace the floor.

## HEADACHE TRIGGERS

The most consistent triggers of headache in cluster headache are alcohol and daytime napping. When a headache is triggered by alcohol, it typically occurs 30–45 minutes after ingestion of even a small quantity of alcohol. The occurrence of episodes of headaches has been related to the lengthening and shortening of days in spring and fall, respectively.

## PATIENT PROFILE

John R. Graham, my mentor in headache, has described cluster headache as the *leonine mouse syndrome*.[3] This refers to the husky appearance of many of these patients and their leonine facial features: ruddy complexion, deep furrows, and prominent eyebrows. In contrast to this very masculine appearance stands an often timid personality, with increased dependency needs. Cluster-headache patients also tend to smoke and drink excessively, which may account for their increased incidence of coronary artery disease, peptic ulcer disease, and cancer.

## REFERENCES

1. D'Alessandro R, Gamberini G, Benassi G, et al. Cluster headache in the Republic of San Marino. Cephalalgia 1986;6:159–162.
2. Kudrow L. Cluster Headache. New York: Oxford University Press, 1980.
3. Graham JR. Cluster headache. Headache 1972;11: 175–185.

# CHAPTER TWENTY-THREE

# Treatment of Cluster Headache

Apart from instructing patients to avoid alcohol and daytime napping during episodes, treatment of cluster headache is pharmacologic. The pharmacologic treatment can be divided into abortive and preventive. Generally, both forms of treatment are applied at the same time, although the emphasis is on preventive treatment because of the high frequency of occurrence of the headaches. Four medications—methysergide (Sansert),[1] verapamil (Isoptin),[2] prednisone (Deltasone),[1] and lithium (Lithobid)[1]—are effective in the preventive treatment of cluster headache. The three medications that are effective in aborting the headaches of cluster headache are sublingual ergotamine (Ergostat),[3] inhaled oxygen,[3] and suma-

**Table 23-1. Medications effective in the treatment of cluster headache**

Abortive treatment
    Ergotamine by sublingual tablet
    Oxygen by inhalation
    Sumatriptan by subcutaneous injection
Preventive treatment
    Methysergide
    Verapamil
    Prednisone
    Lithium

triptan given by subcutaneous injection (Imitrex)[4] (Table 23-1).

## ABORTIVE TREATMENT

### Ergotamine

The sublingual ergotamine tablet contains 2 mg of the medication. It aborts at least 7 out of 10 headaches in 70% of patients, mostly within 10–12 minutes of treatment.[3] The most common side effects are nausea, leg cramps, and a bad aftertaste. Ergotamine is contraindicated in uncontrolled hypertension and coronary artery disease.

## Oxygen

Inhalation of 100% oxygen is somewhat more effective than ergotamine. It is inhaled through a face mask at a rate of 8–10 liters per minute for 15 minutes at the onset of the headache. It aborts at least 7 out of 10 headaches in 82% of patients—in more than half within 6 minutes of treatment.[3] There are no side effects or contraindications to the use of oxygen.

## Sumatriptan

Sumatriptan, in a dose of 6 mg subcutaneously, aborts 74% of cluster headaches within 15 minutes of treatment.[4] A hot, tight, or tingling sensation—generally in the upper chest, anterior neck, and face—and lightheadedness are its most common side effects. As with ergotamine, the medication is contraindicated in uncontrolled hypertension and coronary artery disease.

## PREVENTIVE TREATMENT

## Methysergide

Methysergide is the least effective medication used for preventing cluster headache. In a dose of 8 mg

**Table 23-2. Efficacy of preventive medications in cluster headache**

| Medication | In patients experiencing episodic cluster headache (%) | In patients experiencing chronic cluster headache (%) |
|---|---|---|
| Methysergide[a] | 53 | 7 |
| Verapamil[b] | 73 | 60 |
| Prednisone[a] | 77 | 40 |
| Lithium[a] | — | 87 |

[a]L Kudrow. Comparative Results of Prednisone, Methysergide, and Lithium Therapy in Cluster Headache. In R Greene (ed), Current Concepts in Migraine Research. New York: Raven, 1978;159–163.
[b]IJ Gabai, ELH Spierings. Prophylactic treatment of cluster headache with verapamil. Headache 1989;29:167–168.

per day, methysergide has an efficacy of 53% in episodic cluster headache and 7% in chronic cluster headache (Table 23-2).[1] Efficacy is defined as a reduction in headache frequency of at least 75%. Common side effects of methysergide are nausea and indigestion. With long-term use, methysergide can cause fibrotic conditions. This, in combination with methysergide's low efficacy, make it a useless medication in chronic cluster headache. Methysergide is contraindicated in hypertension, vascular disease, valvular heart disease, chronic pulmonary disease, collagen disease, and fibrotic conditions.

## Verapamil

Verapamil, on the other hand, has an efficacy of 73% in episodic cluster headache and 60% in chronic cluster headache.[2] The daily dosage of *sustained-release* verapamil needed to obtain this effect ranged from 240 to 600 mg in episodic cluster headache and from 240 to 1,200 mg in chronic cluster headache. With the use of doses higher than 480 mg per day, an echocardiogram should be performed to rule out heart muscle disease. It is also recommended that an electrocardiogram be performed several days after each dose increase to determine the impact of the medication on atrioventricular conduction. The most commmon side effect of verapamil is constipation. Verapamil is contraindicated in atrioventricular block and sick sinus syndrome.

## Prednisone

When prednisone is used for the preventive treatment of cluster headache, it is usually given in a course of 3–4 weeks. The initial dose is 40–60 mg per day, which is maintained for 3–5 days. Subsequently, the dose is gradually decreased by 5 mg every 2 days. Prednisone has an efficacy of 77% in preventing episodic cluster headache and 40% in chronic cluster headache.[1] Potential side effects are stomach pain, fluid retention, and insomnia. The medication is contraindicated in hypertension, diabetes mellitus, infectious illness, peptic ulcer disease, and diverticulosis.

## Lithium

Lithium is particularly effective in preventing chronic cluster headache, with an efficacy of 87%.[1] The therapeutic dose generally lies between 600 and 1,200 mg per day. Lithium is contraindicated in electrolyte imbalance and when sodium restriction or diuretic therapy is required. In the latter conditions, lithium toxicity easily develops as a result of increased tubular reabsorption of the medication, which leads to symptoms ranging from tremor to convulsions. Common side effects of the medication are nausea, indigestion, and diarrhea. These symptoms, however, often respond rapidly to a slight lowering of the dose. The maintenance dose of lithium in the treatment of cluster headache does *not* depend on the serum level. It is advisable to keep the serum level below 1.5 mEq per liter, however, and to determine it regularly, together with the serum electrolyte levels and kidney and thyroid functions.

# REFERENCES

1. Kudrow L. Comparative Results of Prednisone, Methysergide, and Lithium Therapy in Cluster Headache. In R Greene (ed), Current Concepts in Migraine Research. New York: Raven, 1978; 159–163.
2. Gabai IJ, Spierings ELH. Prophylactic treatment of cluster headache with verapamil. Headache 1989; 29:167–168.
3. Kudrow L. Response of cluster headache attacks to oxygen inhalation. Headache 1981;12:1–4.
4. Sumatriptan Cluster Headache Study Group. Treatment of acute cluster headache with sumatriptan. N Engl J Med 1991;325:322–326.

# Paroxysmal Hemicrania

An 80-year-old woman has had headaches for 1½–2 years. The headaches have occurred daily since their onset. They occur four to 10 times per day and last for 5–15 minutes. The headaches are very severe and very sharp. They begin and disappear quickly. The headaches wake her out of sleep at night three times per week on average. They are located on the right in the frontotemporal area. The headaches are associated with a warm feeling in the right forehead, whereas her nose feels cold. The headaches are not brought on by anything in particular, and nothing makes them better.

Paroxysmal hemicrania is a variant of cluster headache that is rare but easy to diagnose and treat.[1] It consists of severe unilateral headaches similar to cluster headache, but the headaches are shorter in duration and occur more frequently. The headaches last from 10 to 30 minutes and occur five to 15 times per day. They often occur like clockwork every 2 hours during the day and at night. The headaches occur in episodes with remissions (i.e., episodic) or daily for years (i.e., chronic), as in the patient described in the preceding case study.

The prevalence of paroxysmal hemicrania has been estimated at 2% of that of cluster headache.[2] Women seem to be affected two or three times more frequently than men. The age of onset for almost half of the patients is in the second or third decade of life.

The headaches of paroxysmal hemicrania are *totally* relieved by preventive treatment with indomethacin (Indocin). Generally, the dosage required is 25 mg four times per day or 75 mg of sustained-release indomethacin twice daily. The beneficial effect is usually apparent within 2–5 days of treatment. Indomethacin is contraindicated in peptic ulcer disease and bleeding disorders. When indomethacin is contraindicated, the condition should be treated, as is cluster headache, with verapamil (Isoptin).

# REFERENCE

1. Spierings ELH. Episodic and chronic paroxysmal hemicrania. Clin J Pain 1992;8:44–48.
2. Antonaci F, Sjaastad O. Chronic paroxysmal hemicrania (CPH): a review of the clinical manifestations. Headache 1988;29:648–656.

# CHAPTER TWENTY-FIVE

# Idiopathic Stabbing Headache

A 36-year-old woman has had two bouts of very severe headaches. One bout occurred 1 year ago and the other 2 weeks ago. The first bout lasted for 1 week and the second one for 3 days. During the bouts, the headaches occurred daily. On the first day, they occurred 10 times, after which they gradually decreased in frequency. The headaches were like explosions in the head that lasted for seconds. They were located in the left back of the head, which felt bruised afterward.

## PRESENTATION

Idiopathic stabbing headache, also called *jabs and jolts* or *ice pick–like pains*, are sharp pains in the head that last for a few seconds. They are often so intense that they make the patient grab his or her head when they occur. They begin instantaneously and are sometimes followed by an after-pain, or bruised feeling, which can last for some minutes.

When the pains of idiopathic stabbing headache occur by themselves, the condition has been referred to as *jabs and jolts syndrome*.[1] An episodic and chronic form of this syndrome are distinguished (similar to cluster headache and paroxysmal hemicrania). The preceding case study illustrates the episodic form of the condition. The following case study illustrates the chronic form of idiopathic stabbing headache.

---

An 84-year-old woman has had headaches almost daily for the last year. The headaches began without apparent reason. The pain is shooting in nature and lasts for seconds. The headaches are not located in any particular part of the head. They are so intense that they make her grab her head whenever they occur.

---

The pains of idiopathic stabbing headache can either occur by themselves or in association with other headaches, such as migraine or cluster headache. Their association with these other headache conditions has led to the notion that they are also vascular.

## TREATMENT

In apparent support of the theory that the pains of idiopathic stabbing headache are vascular in nature, they tend to respond to preventive treatment with a vasoconstrictor, such as ergotamine. They also respond to indomethacin (Indocin), although usually the response is only partial. Generally, treatment is indicated only when the pains occur very frequently (i.e., daily and many times per day). I have seen a patient who counted as many as 370 jabs in a single day. He obtained partial relief from these daily headaches with ergotamine, 2–4 mg per day, and complete relief from sustained-release indomethacin, 75 mg twice daily.

## REFERENCE

1. Spierings ELH. Episodic and chronic jabs and jolts syndrome. Headache Q 1990;1:299–302.

# CHAPTER TWENTY-SIX

# Hemicrania Continua

A 48-year-old woman has had headaches since her late teens. Initially, the headaches occurred twice per month and were relieved by a nonprescription analgesic. They gradually increased in frequency and have occurred daily for 2–3 years. The headaches are present on awakening in the morning and do not have a particular diurnal pattern. They do not wake her out of sleep at night. The headaches are located on the right, in the eye, the forehead, the side of the head, and the back of the neck. They are steady, viselike, and mostly moderate in intensity. The headaches are not associated with nausea, vomiting, photophobia, or phonophobia. Bending over makes them worse, and lying down makes the headaches somewhat better. They are also worse with menstrual periods. Her neck and shoulder muscles are tight and sore on the right, and there is some soreness also in the right upper arm. She takes 1,000–1,500 mg of aspirin per day with 40% relief of the headaches. On indomethacin, 25 mg four times per day, she is virtually headache-free.

## PRESENTATION

Hemicrania continua is a form of chronic daily headache, but it must be differentiated from that condition because of its treatment.[1] As with paroxysmal hemicrania, it is a condition with an absolute response to indomethacin. As with cluster headache and paroxysmal hemicrania, it is a unilateral headache syndrome with fixed lateralization (i.e., the headaches *always* occur on the same side of the head). However, whereas cluster headache and paroxysmal hemicrania have typical clinical presentations in terms of the frequency and duration of the headaches, hemicrania continua does not. Therefore, it is *impossible* to diagnose the condition solely on its clinical presentation: Diagnosis also requires the response to indomethacin.

CHRONIC HEADACHE | *26. Hemicrania Continua* **223**

## TREATMENT

Hemicrania continua that is resistant to indomethacin (as has been suggested[2]) does not exist. However, many patients with continuous unilateral headaches with fixed lateralization do not respond to indomethacin. The key in the history is how the headaches respond to aspirin, which seems to predict an absolute response to indomethacin. This feature led to the identification of both paroxysmal hemicrania and hemicrania continua as indomethacin-responsive headache syndromes.

## REFERENCES

1. Sjaastad O, Spierings ELH. "Hemicrania continua": another headache absolutely responsive to indomethacin. Cephalalgia 1984;4:65–70.
2. Kuritzky A. Indomethacin-resistant hemicrania continua. Cephalalgia 1992;12:57–59.

# Index

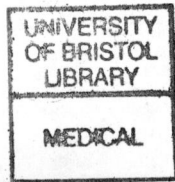

# Bad Blood

### Lily Hayden

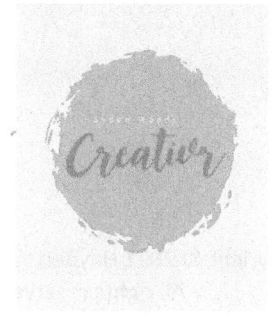